MIND
OVER
MOOD

MIND OVER MOOD

Change How You Feel by Changing the Way You Think

Dennis Greenberger, Ph.D.
Christine A. Padesky, Ph.D.

Foreword by Aaron T. Beck

THE GUILFORD PRESS
New York   London

© 1995 The Guilford Press
A Division of Guilford Publications, Inc.
72 Spring Street, New York, NY 10012

Printed in the United States of America

This book is printed on acid-free paper.

Last digit is print number: 19 18 17 16 15 14 13

Library of Congress Cataloging-in-Publication Data

Greenberger, Dennis.
    Mind over mood : change how you feel by changing the way you think
/ by Dennis Greenberger, Christine A. Padesky; foreword by Aaron T. Beck
      p. cm.
    ISBN 0–89862–128–3
    1. Cognitive therapy—Popular works. 2. Affective disorders
—Treatments. I. Padesky, Christine A. II. Title.
RC489.C63G743 1996
616.89′142—dc20   96-36532
                                                        CIP

Designed and formatted by
KP Company
Brooklyn, NY

Originally published as *Mind Over Mood:
A Cognitive Therapy Treatment Manual for Clients.*

Foreword

Only rarely does a book come along that can truly change your life. *Mind Over Mood* is such a book. Greenberger and Padesky have distilled the wisdom and science of psychotherapy and written an easily understandable manual for change. This book will be read, reread, and recommended to others by therapists, patients, and people seeking to improve their lives.

When I first began developing cognitive therapy in the late 1950s, I had no idea that it would become one of the most successful and widely practiced psychotherapies in the world. Originally, this therapy was designed to help people overcome depression. Our positive results in treating depression were followed by widespread interest in cognitive therapy. Today, cognitive therapy is the fastest-growing form of psychotherapy, in large part because the treatment has been shown to be effective and often rapid in numerous controlled trials.

In the past several decades, cognitive therapy has been successfully used to help patients with depression, panic disorder, phobias, anxiety, anger, stress-related disorders, relationship problems, drug and alcohol abuse, eating disorders, and most of the other difficulties that bring people to therapy. This book teaches readers the central principles that have made this therapy successful for all these problems.

Mind Over Mood will prove to be a significant milestone in the evolution of cognitive therapy. Never before have the nuts and bolts of cognitive therapy been spelled out so explicitly in a step-by-step fashion for the lay public. Greenberger and Padesky generously provide the guiding questions, hints and reminders, and worksheets that they have developed in their own clinical practices, which can be both vehicle and road map for people seeking to make fundamental changes in their life. This is a rare and special book that can easily be used for self-help or as an adjunct to therapy.

Greenberger and Padesky have been students, colleagues, and friends of mine for many years. Together, they have a unique blend of talent, experience, and education that have helped bring this book to fruition. Dennis Greenberger has been an innovator in the application of cognitive therapy in inpatient settings. His inpatient work has given him special expertise working with patients with great life challenges, including highly suicidal patients. In addition, Dr. Greenberger has been visionary in anticipating directions for the future growth of cognitive therapy. He is always eager to make cognitive therapy more widely available and accessible to therapists and the public alike. Dr. Greenberger is a talented therapist, skilled teacher, and accomplished program developer.

Christine Padesky and I have worked together since 1982, teaching cognitive therapy to thousands of therapists worldwide. After hundreds of hours of conversations together, she understands cognitive therapy better than almost any other therapist. I have observed and admire the warmth, clarity, and focus she brings to her relationships with clients. Dr. Padesky founded the Center for Cognitive Therapy in Newport Beach, California, in 1983. It has become the major cognitive therapy training center for therapists in the western United States. As a workshop instructor, she has taught cognitive therapy to more therapists than any other person except me. She is well-respected by her colleagues and in 1992 was voted president-elect of the International Association for Cognitive Psychotherapy.

Dr. Greenberger's vision and innovation combined with Dr. Padesky's superb abilities as a teacher and therapist are melded in this exemplary book. In the same way that *Cognitive Therapy of Depression*, which I cowrote with John Rush, Brian Shaw, and Gary Emery (New York: Guilford Press, 1979), revolutionized how therapy was conducted, *Mind Over Mood* sets a standard for how cognitive therapy will be utilized by patients. Its explicit instructions will help patients adhere more closely to cognitive therapy principles and consequently improve the quality of their therapy. *Mind Over Mood* is an effective tool that puts cognitive therapy in the hands of the reader.

AARON T. BECK M.D.
University Professor of Psychiatry
University of Pennsylvania

Acknowledgments

We are indebted to Aaron T. Beck for his pioneering development of cognitive therapy. His work is the foundation and inspiration for all the ideas in *Mind Over Mood*. As mentor, colleague, and friend, he helped define both of our careers as psychologists. He actively supported this project and generously provided critical feedback to improve the book's value for clients. We hope this manual is consistent with his vision of cognitive therapy and that it provides clear guidance so people can help themselves—a central commitment of his own work he has passed along to us.

Kathleen A. Mooney critiqued early versions of this book and provided detailed feedback on every chapter. Her gentle honesty, unending enthusiasm, and creativity as a skilled cognitive therapist, as well as her editorial and visual design expertise substantially enhanced the content and format of the book.

Kitty Moore offered valuable editorial assistance at critical junctures in the book's development. From early creative planning sessions to the delivery of the book into production, she has been a strong advocate for *Mind Over Mood* and a source of encouragement for us. In fact, everyone with whom we worked at Guilford consistently reflected the professionalism, intelligence, and integrity that make Guilford a leader in mental health publishing. We extend special appreciation to Seymour Weingarten, the Editor-in Chief, for sharing our vision, and to the Managing Editor, Rowena Howells, for giving our book special personal attention.

Special thanks to Jan Janssen for typing innumerable drafts and revisions, often under deadline. She has a wonderful ability to maintain cheerfulness and grace under all working conditions.

Rose Mooney's feedback on an early draft led to restructuring of several chapters to improve readability. She served as our image of the ideal thoughtful reader as we were writing this book.

The cognitive therapy community contributed to this book in innumerable ways. Cognitive therapists who read early drafts and provided valuable suggestions include Judy Beck, Don Meichenbaum, Jacqueline Persons, Paul Salkovskis, James Shenk, and Jesse Wright. Several agreed to take the lead and initiate research projects to evaluate the impact of this manual on clinical outcomes: Gillian Butler and Helen Kennerley at Oxford University, Cary Glass at Kaiser Permanente, Jan Scott at the University of Newcastle-upon-Tyne, and Michael Thase at Western Psychiatric Institute in Pittsburgh. A number of people used drafts of this manuscript in inpatient hospitals and provided early support for our ideas: Joe Arnold, China Dusk, Jennifer Fog-Toops, Martin Brenner, Linda Donelson, and Judy House.

These and other cognitive therapists taught us through their experience, insights, and clinical innovations. Additional people deserving special recognition in this category include David Clark, Denise Davis, Gary Emery, Melanie Fennell, Barbara Fleming, Art Freemen, Steve Hollon, Robin Jarrett, Bruce Liese, Jim Pretzer, and Jeff Young. Weekly case consultations at the Center for Cognitive Therapy, Newport Beach with Diane Cornsweet, Kathleen Mooney, Marcia Mordkin, Marlyn Osborn, Karen Simon, Gail Simpson, Steve Sultanoff, and Linda Wise advanced Christine Padesky's skill and knowledge during the course of writing this book.

We are fortunate to have so many creative colleagues. We are also grateful that our own collaborative process in writing this book was such a pleasure; our work was accompanied by laughter and discovery. We literally wrote each page together, a process that was labor intensive but led to a text far better than what either of us could have produced alone.

Numerous clients used drafts of *Mind Over Mood* and offered thoughtful feedback. In addition, every client with whom we have worked has asked questions and shared experiences that contributed to our understanding of how people change. Although we are unable to acknowledge you by name, this book is a product of your openness and hard work. You have taught us to be better therapists and we hope your lessons to us are reflected in this book.

D.G. & C.A.P.

On an individual basis,

Thanks to Deidre Greenberger for her warmth and love. Her unwavering faith in me and this project is a source of continuing strength. Her intelligence, humor, spontaneity, curiosity, and wisdom added to this book and to my life. And to Elysa and Alanna Greenberger, the two sweetest blessings in my life.

Dennis Greenberger

I extend special appreciation to all the therapists who have attended my training programs and workshops, especially participants in the Intensive Training Program, annual Winter Workshop, and Camp Cognitive Therapy I and II. Your wonderful questions and dedication to becoming excellent cognitive therapists inspire me to try to write clearer explanations of how cognitive therapy is done. Hopefully, this book will show many people how to use cognitive therapy to improve their moods and their lives.

Christine A. Padesky

Contents

Prologue

An oyster creates a pearl out of a grain of sand. The grain of sand is an irritant to the oyster. In response to the discomfort, the oyster creates a smooth, protective coating that encases the sand and provides relief. The result is a beautiful pearl.

For an oyster, an irritant becomes the seed for something new. Similarly, *Mind Over Mood* will help you develop something valuable from your current discomfort. The skills taught in this book will help you feel better and will continue to have value in your life long after your original problems are gone.

HOW WILL THIS BOOK HELP YOU?

Mind Over Mood teaches methods that have been shown to be helpful with mood problems such as depression, anxiety, anger, panic, jealousy, guilt, and shame. The strategies described in this book can also help you solve relationship problems, handle stress better, improve your self-esteem, become less fearful and more confident. Further, these strategies can help you if you are struggling to maintain sobriety or to live your life without drugs. *Mind Over Mood* provides structure that can help you proceed efficiently and rapidly in making changes.

The ideas in this book come from cognitive therapy, one of today's most successful forms of psychotherapy. "Cognitive" means "thought processes" as well as "knowledge" or "perception." Cognitive therapists emphasize examination of the thoughts and beliefs connected to our moods, behaviors, physical experiences, and to the events in our lives. A central idea in cognitive therapy is that our *perception* of an event or experience powerfully affects our emotional, behavioral, and physiological responses to it.

For example, if we are standing in line at the grocery store and think, "This will take awhile, I may as well just relax," we are likely to feel calm. Our body stays relaxed, and we may start a conversation with someone standing nearby or pick up a magazine. However, if we think, "This place is poorly managed. It's not fair to have such a long line," we may feel angry. Our body is tense or fidgety, and we may spend our time looking at our watch or grumbling to the clerk.

Mind Over Mood teaches you to identify your thoughts, moods, behaviors, and physical reactions in small situations as well as during major events in your life. You learn to test the meaning and usefulness of various thoughts you have during the day and to change the thinking patterns that keep you locked into dysfunctional moods, behaviors, or relationship interactions. In addition, you learn how to make changes in your life when your thoughts are alerting you to problems that need to be solved.

HOW TO USE THIS BOOK

This book is different from most books you read. *Mind Over Mood* teaches you skills that are necessary to make fundamental changes in your moods, behaviors, and relationships. Therefore, it is important for you to complete the exercises in each chapter. If you move too quickly through the book without giving yourself adequate time to practice the skills taught, you will not learn how to apply the skills to your own problems. Even some of the skills that look easy can be more complicated than they seem when you actually try to do them.

If a therapist or other professional recommended this book to you, he or she may suggest that you read the chapters in a different order than printed here. While each chapter adds to your knowledge and abilities, some people will not need to use every chapter. Each chapter includes exercises to guide discovery of important learning points. Additional copies of the exercise worksheets can be found in the Appendix at the end of the book so that you can duplicate and use them whenever you think they might help.

We hope that, like many people who have learned the methods taught in this book, you will look back at the initial discomfort that led you to *Mind Over Mood* as a "blessing in disguise," because it provided you the opportunity and motivation to develop pearls of perspective that will help you enjoy the rest of your life more fully.

CHAPTER 1

Understanding Your Problems

BEN: *I hate getting old.*

One afternoon a therapist received a telephone call from Sylvie, a 68-year-old woman who was concerned about her husband, Ben. She had read an article in *Reader's Digest* about depression and wondered if that was what was troubling him. For the past six months, Ben had complained constantly about feeling tired, yet Sylvie would hear him pacing around the living room at three in the morning, unable to sleep. In addition, she said he was not as warm toward her, he was often irritable, and he showed no interest in golfing or visiting friends. After an annual medical checkup cleared Ben of any physical problems, Ben complained to his wife, "I hate getting old, it feels lousy."

The therapist asked to talk with Ben on the phone, and Ben reluctantly came on the line. He told the therapist not to take it personally, but he didn't think much of "head doctors" and didn't want to see the therapist because he wasn't crazy, just old. "You wouldn't be happy either if you were 71 and ached all over!" He said he would go to one appointment just to satisfy Sylvie, but he hoped it wouldn't cost too much because he was sure it wouldn't help.

How we understand our problems has an effect on how we cope. Ben thought his sleep problems, tiredness, irritability, and lack of interest in golfing with friends were normal parts of growing older. Growing old was something Ben couldn't change, so he didn't expect anything could help him feel better.

When people see a therapist about problems, the first first thing the therapist does is to encourage understanding the problems. The therapist asks questions about the five aspects of life shown in Figure 1.1: thoughts

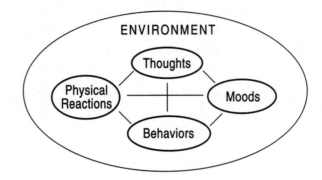

FIGURE 1.1. Five aspects of your life experiences. © 1986 Center for Cognitive Therapy, Newport Beach, CA.

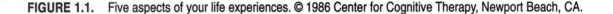

(beliefs, images, memories), moods, behaviors, physical reactions, and environment (past and present). Notice that the five areas are interconnected. The connecting lines show that each different aspect of a person's life influences all the others. For example, changes in our behavior influence how we think and also how we feel (both physically and emotionally). Behavior changes can also change our environment. Likewise, changes in our thinking affect our behavior, mood, physical reactions, and can lead to changes in our social environment. Understanding how these five parts of our lives interact can help us understand our problems.

Let's look in on Ben and his therapist at their first meeting to see what we can learn to help us understand Ben's problems. In the waiting room, the therapist was immediately struck by the difference in Sylvie's and Ben's appearance. In a rose-colored skirt with a coordinating floral blouse, earrings, and shoes, Sylvie had dressed herself carefully for the meeting. She sat upright in her chair and greeted the therapist with an expectant smile and bright, eager eyes. In contrast, Ben was slumped slightly in his chair, and although he was neatly dressed in golf slacks and shirt, he had a slight stubble on the left side of his chin. His eyes were dull and surrounded by the dark circles of fatigue. He stood up stiffly and slowly to greet the therapist, saying grimly, "Well, you got me for an hour."

As the therapist gently questioned Ben over the next 30 minutes, his story slowly unfolded. With each question he sighed deeply and then responded flatly. Ben had been a postal carrier for 35 years, walking the same community for the last 14 of those years. After his retirement, he had become a regular golfer, playing four times a week with three retired friends. Ben also liked to putter in the garage, working on house projects and repairing bicycles for his eight young grandchildren and their friends. He regularly gave financial advice to his three children and felt proud to have a good relationship with each of them.

Eighteen months earlier, Sylvie had been diagnosed with breast cancer. Her cancer had been detected early, and she had recovered well after surgery and chemotherapy, with no further signs of cancer. Ben became teary as he talked about her illness: "I thought I'd lose her and didn't know what I'd do." As he said this, Sylvie jumped in quickly, patting Ben on the arm, "But I'm OK, dear. Everything turned out OK." Ben swallowed hard and nodded his head.

While Sylvie was undergoing cancer treatment, one of Ben's golfing partners, Louie, became suddenly ill with pneumonia and died. Louie had been Ben's friend for 18 years, and Ben felt his loss deeply. He felt angry that Louie had not gone to the hospital sooner, because early treatment might have saved his life. Sylvie said Ben became obsessed with tracking her cancer treatment appointments after Louie's death. "I think Ben thought he would be responsible for my death if we missed an appointment," said Sylvie. Ben stopped playing golf and devoted himself to Sylvie's care.

"After Sylvie's treatment ended, I knew the relief was only temporary. The rest of my life will be filled with illness and death. I feel half dead already. A young person like yourself can't understand this." Ben sighed. "It's just as well. What use am I anyway? The grandkids fix their own bikes now. My sons have a financial planner, and Sylvie would probably have more fun if I wasn't dragging her down. I don't know what's worse—to die or to live and be left all alone because all your friends are dead."

After hearing Ben's story and reviewing his physician's report, which cleared Ben of any physical problems, it was clear to the therapist that he was indeed depressed. He was experiencing physical symptoms (insomnia, appetite loss, fatigue), behavior changes (he had stopped doing activities, he was avoiding friends), mood changes (sadness, irritability, guilt), and a thinking style (negative, self-critical, and pessimistic) consistent with depression. As is often the case with depression, Ben had experienced a number of losses and stresses in the preceding two years (Sylvie's cancer, Louie's death, and a reduction in his perception of how much his children and grandchildren needed him).

Although Ben was skeptical that therapy could help, with Sylvie's encouragement he agreed to go to three more sessions before deciding whether to go on with it or not.

UNDERSTANDING BEN'S PROBLEMS

During their second meeting, Ben's therapist helped Ben list his personal changes using the model in Figure 1.1. Only then did Ben notice that a number of *environmental* changes and events in his life (Sylvie's cancer, Louie's death) had led to *behavior* changes (the end of his regular golf foursome, extra trips to the hospital for Sylvie's cancer treatment). In addition, he began to *think* differently about himself and his life ("Everyone I care about is dying," "My children and grandchildren no longer need me") and feel worse both *emotionally* (irritable, sad) and *physically* (tired, more trouble sleeping).

Ben could see how each of the five life aspects influenced the other four, pulling him deeper into his sad mood. For example, as a result of thinking "All my friends will die soon because we're getting old" (thought change), Ben stopped calling them on the phone (behavior change). As Ben became more isolated from his friends, he began to feel lonely and sad (mood change), and his inactivity contributed to making him feel tired (physical change). Since he no longer called his friends or did things with them, many of them stopped calling him (social environment change). Over time, these interacting forces dragged Ben into a downward spiral of depression.

At first, when Ben's therapist pointed out this pattern, Ben was discouraged: "It's hopeless, then—each of these things will just get worse and worse until I die!" The therapist pointed out that since each of the five areas of his life was connected to the other four, small improvements in any of the areas could contribute to positive change in the other four. Therapy could help Ben figure out what small changes would make him feel better.

Ben is one of four people you will meet in this chapter whom we will follow throughout this book. These four people are representative of the kinds of people who are often helped by the methods described in *Mind Over Mood*. To protect confidentiality, identifying information has been changed and some descriptive information is a composite of several clients. However, all the information is consistent with our experiences as therapists helping people with these types of problems.

MARISSA: *My life doesn't seem worth living.*

Marissa was also depressed. During her first meeting with her therapist, she confided that she was increasingly upset and was beginning to feel out of control. She said that her depression had become worse over the previous six months. This depression frightened her because she had been seriously depressed twice before—once when she was 18 years old and again at age 25—and had made suicide attempts during each episode. With tears in her eyes, she rolled up her sleeve and showed the scars on her wrist from her first suicide attempt.

Marissa said that she had been sexually molested by her father between the ages of 6 and 14. At age 14 her parents divorced. By this time, Marissa already thought of herself in negative terms. "I decided I must be bad for my father to hurt me like he did. I was afraid to get close to other kids for fear they would know what had happened to me; I was afraid of adults because I thought they would hurt me."

Given her history of low self-esteem, it is not surprising that Marissa agreed to marry her first boyfriend, Carl. She and Carl were married at age 17 when she became pregnant and divorced three years later, shortly after the birth of her second child. Her second marriage, at age 23, lasted only two years. Both of her husbands were alcoholic and physically abusive.

Despite being depressed for 18 months following her second divorce, Marissa emerged from this desperate period in her life feeling stronger. She decided that she could care for her children better on her own without her ex-husband. She began working and supporting her children with the assistance of neighborhood day care. She was a loving mother to her children and was proud of them. The older child, now age 18, was beginning community college and the younger one was in high school.

Now, at age 36, Marissa was personnel assistant in a manufacturing plant. Despite her successes as a working mother, Marissa was self-critical. During the initial meeting she made minimal eye contact, staring at her hands in her lap. She spoke in a low monotone and did not smile. Her eyes welled up with tears on several occasions as she talked about how "worthless" she was and how bleak her future would be. "I've been thinking more and more about killing myself. The kids are old enough to take care of themselves. My pain will never end. Death is the only way out."

In response to questions about her life and what made it so painful to her, Marissa described intense sadness all day long. As her depression became worse over the last six months, Marissa found it increasingly difficult to work and concentrate on her job. She had been given two verbal warnings and a written notice from her supervisor regarding the timeliness, quality, and quantity of her work. She found herself more and more tired and less and less motivated.

At home, Marissa just wanted to be left alone. She would not answer the phone or talk with family or friends. She prepared minimal meals for her children and then closed herself in her room, watching television until she fell asleep.

At the first meeting, Marissa was not particularly hopeful that cognitive therapy would help her, but she had promised her family physician that she would give it a try. She felt that she had a limited number of choices and that if this treatment didn't work, suicide would be her only remaining option. Needless to say, the therapist was very concerned about Marissa and wanted to help her begin to feel better as soon as possible. The therapist referred her to a psychiatrist for a consultation to see if medication might help her, even though she had been helped only minimally by antidepressants in the past. The next appointment was set for only a few days later so that Marissa would not have to wait long to begin.

UNDERSTANDING MARISSA'S PROBLEMS

If we use the five-part model in Figure 1.1 to understand Marissa's depression, we see some similarities between Marissa and Ben in thinking patterns, mood, behavior, and physical experiences. And yet the social environment part of Marissa's depression began back in her early childhood.

The following list summarizes Marissa's depression.

- *Environmental changes/Life situations*: Sexually molested by father; two alcoholic and abusive husbands; single parent of two teenagers; negative feedback from work supervisor.
- *Physical reactions*: Tired most of the time.
- *Moods*: Depressed.
- *Behaviors*: Difficulty working; isolating self from other people; crying, suicide attempts.
- *Thoughts*: "I'm no good," "I'm a failure," "I'm never going to get better," "My life is hopeless," "I may as well kill myself."

Some people may think Marissa was doomed to depression because of her harsh life experiences. As you will see, this was not true.

LINDA: *My life would be great if I didn't have panic attacks!*

"One of my friends told me there is a new therapy for panic attacks—do you think it would help me?" The phone caller was very direct in her questioning. Her voice was firm and confident as she quizzed the therapist about cognitive therapy. She was equally direct in recounting the recent experiences that had prompted her call. "My name is Linda. I'm 29 years old and, except for a fear of flying in airplanes, I've never had any problems I couldn't handle myself. I'm a marketing supervisor for the phone company and have always loved my job—until two months ago, that is. Two months ago I was promoted to regional supervisor. Now I'll have to fly all over the West Coast and I find myself breaking into cold sweats whenever I think about it. I was thinking of turning down the promotion when my friend told me to call you first. Can you help?"

Linda arrived early for her first appointment with her briefcase and a notebook, ready to begin learning what to do. She had been afraid of flying her entire life, a fear she suspected she learned from her mother, who avoided airplanes. Her panic attacks were more recent and had actually preceded the job promotion.

Linda recalled that her first panic attack had been eight months earlier when she noticed her heart pounding during Saturday shopping at the grocery store. She couldn't understand why this was happening and became quite frightened. This was the first time she broke into a sweat from fear. At the time she thought she was having a heart attack, but a visit to the hospital emergency room assured her that she had no physical problems.

Linda continued to have panic attacks once or twice a month until the recent job promotion. Since her promotion she had been gripped by fear several times a week. Her heart would race, she would break into a sweat, and would find herself struggling to breathe. The panicky feeling would "just come out of the blue—even at home" and last for a few minutes until it disappeared almost as fast as it had come.

"I support myself, I've managed to buy a small condo, I have good friends and a supportive family, I don't drink or use drugs, I've always lived a good life—why is this happening to me?" Linda had in fact led a happy, hard-working and balanced life. Her only major trauma had been the death of her father a year earlier. She missed him, yet took comfort from her relationship with her mother and two brothers who lived nearby. Although her job required hard work, Linda seemed to enjoy the pressure and manage her stress well.

Why was Linda suffering from panic attacks? In the chapters that follow, you will watch Linda as she learned to discover and interpret the causes of her panic attacks. By learning more about her physical reactions, thoughts, and behaviors, Linda not only learned to overcome her panic, she also became a frequent flyer for the phone company.

UNDERSTANDING LINDA'S PROBLEMS

Linda had panic attacks and also a fear of flying in airplanes, both anxiety-related problems. Can the model in Figure 1.1 be used to understand anxiety? Notice how the five areas summarize Linda's experiences:

- *Environmental changes/Life situations*: Death of father; job promotion.
- *Physical reactions*: Cold sweats; pounding heart; breathing difficulty.
- *Moods*: Fear; panic.
- *Behaviors*: Avoiding flying; may relinquish job promotion.
- *Thoughts*: "I'm having a heart attack," "Something bad will happen if I fly."

As you can see, the five-part model can help describe anxiety as well as depression. Notice some of the differences between anxiety and depression. Physical changes associated with depression often involve a slowing down—trouble sleeping (Ben) and feeling tired (Ben and Marissa)—whereas anxiety is usually marked by a speeding up of the physical—pounding heart, increased sweating (Linda). With depression, people find it difficult to do things and often withdraw from people. Linda describes enjoying people and her job, but she avoids specific things that make her anxious. Avoidance is characteristic of anxiety.

Finally, thinking is quite different in the states of depression and anxiety. Ben and Marissa illustrate depressed thinking, which tends to be negative, hopeless, and self-critical. Linda's thinking is more catastrophic ("I'm having a heart attack") and involves worry about specific future events (an airplane flight), which is more typical of anxiety. Rather than thinking of herself in generally negative terms, as people do when depressed, Linda sees herself as vulnerable in a few specific situations, a view more typical of anxiety. Chapters 10, 11, and 12 further summarize the distinguishing characteristics of different moods.

VIC: *Help me be more perfect.*

Vic, a 49-year-old marketing executive, began therapy three years after acknowledging his alcoholism and joining Alcoholics Anonymous (AA). Over six feet tall and athletically built, Vic arrived for his first appointment neatly dressed in a gray pin-striped suit and a maroon tie. Every part of Vic's appearance was perfect, from his neatly trimmed hair to his highly polished shoes.

Despite frequent urges to drink, Vic had not touched a drop of alcohol in three years. His urge to drink was strongest when he felt sad or nervous. At these times, he thought, "Alcohol will make me feel better and deaden these uncomfortable feelings." His attendance at AA meetings was irregular, and resisting drinking was a struggle.

Vic was subject to periods of depression, during which he saw himself as "no good," "worthless," and "a failure." He was often jumpy and nervous. During his nervous times, Vic worried again and again that he would be fired from his job for poor performance, despite the fact that he consistently received good evaluations and exceeded the company-established job goals. When the phone in his office rang, Vic anticipated that the caller would be his boss, telling him he had been fired. He was surprised and relieved each time this did not happen.

Vic described his 25-year battle with alcohol as a result of lifelong feelings of inadequacy, low self-esteem, and a sense that something "awful" was going to happen to him. When he drank he felt better, stronger, and "in control." Becoming sober had put the spotlight on his deep feelings of worthlessness, anxiety, and poor self-esteem, which the alcohol had covered up.

Early in therapy it became clear that Vic tried to cope with his moods by being a perfectionist. He had been told by his parents, "If you make a mistake, it's bad." "If you're going to do something at all, do it right." Vic had concluded, "If I'm not perfect, then I'm a failure."

Vic grew up with one older brother, Doug, who was a star athlete and straight-A student. As a child, Vic felt that his parents' approval, love, and affection depended on his performance. Although his parents showed their love for Vic in many ways, he never felt that they were as proud of him as they were of Doug. He felt pressured to be the best in school and sports. One year he scored a touchdown in a big football game, yet Vic was disappointed because a teammate scored two touchdowns in the same game. A good performance was not enough for Vic if it was not also the best.

As an adult Vic found it harder and harder to be the best. He juggled the roles of husband, father, and marketing executive, judging his worth by his performance in each of these areas. He rarely felt perfect in any area of his life and consequently worried about how other people evaluated him. If he worked long hours at the office to please his boss, he worried on the drive home that he was letting down his wife and children.

Vic came to therapy looking for ways to feel better about himself and wanting to feel more confident. He also wanted to get help staying sober. At the end of the first session, he told the therapist, with a laugh, "Look, all I want is for you to make me perfect and then I'll be perfectly happy." The therapist suggested to Vic that maybe one goal of therapy should be to help him feel happy with himself as he was, imperfections and all. Vic swallowed hard and tentatively nodded his head.

UNDERSTANDING VIC'S PROBLEMS

Of course, sometimes we have more than one strong mood. Vic was experiencing both depression and anxiety. Using the five-part model, we would expect to find in his case similarities with Ben and Marissa (depression) and also with Linda (anxiety). Making out the list for Vic, we find this to be true.

Environmental changes/Life situations: Three years of sobriety; lifelong pressure (by parents, self) to be the best.

Physical reactions: Occasional insomnia; stomach problems.

Moods: Nervous; frustrated.

Behaviors: Difficulty resisting urges to drink; sometimes avoiding Alcoholics Anonymous meetings; trying to do everything perfectly.

Thoughts: "I'm no good," "I'm worthless, " "I'm a failure," "I'll be fired," "I'm inadequate," "Something awful will happen," "If I make a mistake, I'm no good."

As you can see, Vic's thinking was negative and self-critical (typical of depression) and also involved worry, self-doubt, and catastrophic predictions (typical of anxiety). His physical problems could have been signs of either depression or anxiety. His behavior was more typical of anxiety because Vic was avoiding only particular situations in his life; he was still performing well at work and enjoying his relationships.

EXERCISE: Understanding Your Own Problems

Just as you did for Ben, Marissa, Linda, and Vic, you can begin to understand your own problems by defining what you are experiencing in these five areas of your life: environment, physical reactions, moods, behaviors, and thoughts. On Worksheet 1.1, describe any recent changes or long-term problems you have experienced in each of these areas. If you have difficulty filling out Worksheet 1.1, ask yourself the questions in the "Helpful Hints" box that follows.

WORKSHEET 1.1: Understanding My Problems

Environmental changes/Life situations: _____

_____

Physical reactions: _____

_____

Moods: _____

_____

Behaviors: _____

_____

Thoughts: _____

_____

As you will see throughout this book, no matter what changes contribute to your problems (lifelong beliefs, behaviors, physical changes), once you are depressed or anxious or experience some other strong mood, all five aspects of your experience shown in Figure 1.1 are involved. While small changes in all five areas may be necessary to feel better, you will learn that changes in your thinking are often most important if you want to create lasting positive improvements in your life. Chapter 2 will help explain why this is so.

HELPFUL HINTS

If you are having trouble filling out Worksheet 1.1, the following questions will help you:

Environmental changes/Life situations: Have I experienced any recent changes? What have been the most stressful events for me in the past year? 3 years? 5 years? In childhood? Do I experience any long-term or ongoing difficulties (including discrimination or harassment by others)?

Physical reactions: Do I experience any physical symptoms that trouble me, such as changes in energy level, appetite, and sleep, as well as specific symptoms, such as heart rate fluctuations, stomachaches, sweating, dizziness, breathing difficulties, or pain?

Moods: What single words describe my moods (sad, nervous, angry, guilty, ashamed)?

Behaviors: What things do I do that I would like to change or improve? At work? At home? With friends? By myself? Do I avoid situations or people when it might be to my advantage to be involved?

Thoughts: When I have strong moods, what thoughts do I have about myself? Other people? My future? What thoughts interfere with doing the things I would like to do or think I should do? What images or memories come into my mind?

From *Mind Over Mood* by Dennis Greenberger and Christine A. Padesky. © 1995 The Guilford Press.

CHAPTER 1 SUMMARY

- There are five components to any problem: environment, physical, moods, behaviors, and thoughts.

- Each of the five components affects and interacts with the others.

- Small changes in any one area can lead to changes in the other areas.

- Identifying the five components of your own distress can help target areas for change (Worksheet 1.1).

CHAPTER 2

It's the Thought That Counts

In Chapter 1 you learned how thinking, mood, behavior, physical reactions, and environment are all connected to each other. In this chapter you will learn that when you want to feel better, improve your relationships, or change your behavior, your thoughts are often the place to start. This chapter describes how learning more about your thoughts can help you in many areas of your life.

WHAT IS THE THOUGHT/MOOD CONNECTION?

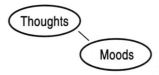

Whenever we experience a mood, there is a thought connected to it which helps define the mood. For example, suppose you are at a party and you have been introduced to Alex. As you talk, Alex never looks at you; in fact, throughout your brief conversation he looks over your shoulder across the room. Following are three different thoughts you might have in this situation. Four moods are listed below each thought. Circle the one mood that you believe would follow each of these interpretations of Alex not looking at you:

THOUGHT: *Alex is rude. He is insulting me by ignoring me.*

Possible moods (circle one):   Irritated   Sad   Nervous   Caring

THOUGHT: *Alex doesn't find me interesting. I bore everybody.*

Possible moods (circle one):   Irritated   Sad   Nervous   Caring

THOUGHT: *Alex seems shy. He's probably too uncomfortable to look at me.*

Possible moods (circle one):   Irritated   Sad   Nervous   Caring

This example illustrates that different thoughts or interpretations of an event can lead to different moods in the same situation. Since moods are often distressing or may lead to behavior with consequences (such as telling Alex he is rude), it is important to identify what you are thinking and to check out the accuracy of your thoughts before acting. For instance, if Alex were shy, it would be inaccurate to think of him as rude and inappropriate to respond with anger or irritation.

Even situations you might think would create the same mood for everyone—such as losing a job—may, in fact, lead to different moods because of different personal beliefs and meanings. For example, one person facing job loss might think, "I'm a failure," and feel depressed. Another person might think, "They have no right to fire me; this is discrimination," and feel angry. A third person might think, "I don't like this, but now is my chance to try out a new job," and feel a mixture of nervousness and anticipation.

Thoughts help define which mood we experience in a given situation. Once a mood is present, it is accompanied by additional thoughts that support and strengthen the mood. For example, angry people think about ways they have been hurt, depressed people think about how unfortunate life has become, and anxious people see danger everywhere. In fact, the stronger our moods, the more extreme our thinking is likely to be.

This does not mean that our thinking is wrong when we experience an intense mood. But when we feel intense moods, we are more likely to distort, discount, or disregard information that contradicts our moods and beliefs. Everyone thinks in these ways sometimes. However, it is helpful to learn to recognize when you are thinking in distorted ways because this understanding provides a first step toward more balanced thinking and mood states. The following example shows how Marissa's depression is supported by distortions in her thinking.

MARISSA: *The thought/mood connection.*

Marissa thinks she is unlovable. This belief seems absolutely true to her. Given her negative experiences with men, she can't even imagine that someone could truly love her. This belief, coupled with her desire to be in a relationship, leads her to feel depressed. When a work colleague, Julio, begins to fall in love with her, she has the following experiences:

- A friend teases her about the frequent phone calls she receives at work from Julio, saying, "I think you have an admirer, Marissa!" Marissa replies, "What do you mean? He doesn't call that often." (*Not noticing positive information*)

- Julio compliments Marissa and she thinks, "He is just saying this to keep up a good work relationship." (*Discounting positive information*)

- When Julio asks to meet her for lunch, Marissa thinks, "I'm probably explaining the work project so poorly that he resents the extra time the project is taking." (*Jumping to a negative conclusion*)

- At lunch, Julio tells Marissa he thinks that they have both been very creative on the project and says he has really enjoyed spending the extra time with her because she is a respectful, thoughtful woman. He goes on to tell her that he finds her attractive. Marissa says, "Oh, lots of the other team members could have done better." (*Discounting positive feedback*)

Since Marissa is convinced that she is unlovable, she ignores or distorts information that counters this conclusion. When she is very depressed or angry or anxious, she is even less likely to hear positive feedback. Ignoring information that doesn't fit our beliefs is something we can learn to change. For Marissa, learning to take in positive information about her attractiveness and lovability may be the start of something wonderful.

WHAT IS THE THOUGHT/BEHAVIOR CONNECTION?

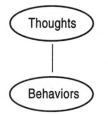

Sometimes our thoughts and behaviors seem quite disconnected—such as when we pour milk into a cup of coffee and then put the cup of coffee into the refrigerator, and carry the milk carton to the table. Despite these occasional lapses in concentration, our thoughts and behaviors are usually closely connected. This is why it is difficult to do more than one or two things at once.

Throughout the day we repeat well-rehearsed behaviors over and over. Perhaps we always give in when someone disagrees with us. We are not aware of the thoughts guiding our behavior because our actions have become routine. However, when we decide to change or learn a new behavior, thoughts can determine whether and how this change occurs.

For example, our expectations affect our behavior. We are more likely to try to do something and succeed if we believe it is possible. For many years, athletes believed it was impossible for humans to run a 4-minute mile. In track events around the world, top milers ran a mile in just over 4 minutes. Then a British miler named Roger Bannister decided to determine what changes he could make in his running style and strategy to break the 4-minute barrier. He believed it was possible to run faster and put many months of effort into changing his running pattern to reach this goal. In 1954 Roger Bannister became the first man to run a mile in less than 4 minutes. His belief that he could succeed contributed to behavior change.

Remarkably, once Bannister broke the record, the best milers from around the world also began to run the mile in under 4 minutes. Unlike Bannister, these runners had not substantially changed their running patterns. What had changed were their thoughts; they now believed it was possible to run this fast and their behavior followed their thoughts. Of course, just knowing it is possible to run fast does not mean everyone can do this. Thinking is not the same as doing. But the more we believe something is possible the more likely we are to attempt it and maybe succeed at it.

"Automatic thoughts" are another type of thought that influences behavior. These are the words and images that pop into our head throughout the day as we are doing things. For example, imagine that you are at a family reunion. The food has just been put out, and some family members go over to the buffet tables to fill their plates while others remain seated and talking. You have been talking with your cousin for 10 minutes. Consider each of the following thoughts and write the behavior that would follow if this were your thought.

THOUGHT	BEHAVIOR
If I don't go now, they'll run out of food.	_____
It's rude to rush to the food tables when we're in the middle of a conversation.	_____
My grandfather looks too unsteady to carry a plate.	_____
My cousin and I are having such a wonderful conversation—I've never met anyone so interesting.	_____

Did your behavior vary depending on the thought you had?

In addition to automatic thoughts, we have deep core beliefs that influence both our automatic thoughts and our behavior patterns. These underlying beliefs are about ourselves ("I'm smart," "I'm weak"), about other people ("People can't be trusted," "Women are strong"), and about life in general ("Good things follow bad," "Change is overwhelming"). How do these underlying beliefs influence our behavior? An example from Ben's life illustrates underlying beliefs at work.

BEN: *The thought/behavior connection.*

After his friend Louie died, Ben cut back on golfing and other activities he shared with his friends. At first, his family thought that avoiding his friends was part of Ben's grief over Louie's death. But as the months passed and Ben refused to get together with friends, his wife, Sylvie, began to suspect that his moods were not the only reason Ben was staying at home.

One morning Sylvie sat down with Ben and asked him why he was not returning his friends' telephone calls. Ben shrugged and said, "What's the point? We're at that age where we're all just dying anyhow." Sylvie felt exasperated. "But you're alive now—do the things you enjoy!" Ben shook his head; Sylvie just didn't understand.

Sylvie really didn't understand, because Ben was not aware of the underlying beliefs guiding his behavior and he couldn't fully explain to her why he had stopped doing activities he used to enjoy. As Ben learned to identify his thoughts, he realized that he was operating according to one of his father's favorite sayings: "Play with your friends when the sun is shining because when the sun begins to set you need to go home alone." When Louie died, Ben decided he had reached the age where death was close at hand. The sun was setting in his own life and so it was time to go home alone.

WHAT IS THE THOUGHT/PHYSICAL REACTIONS CONNECTION?

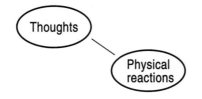

Thoughts also affect our physical reactions. Recall the last time you read an engaging book or magazine article. As your mind imagined the scenes described, your body reacted as well. Imagining a frightening scene can lead to a more rapid heart rate. Imagining a romantic scene can lead to sexual arousal.

Athletes use the powerful link between thoughts and physical reactions. Coaches give their teams inspirational speeches, which they hope will "fire up" the team members and get adrenalin flowing. Olympic swimmers and track stars are often coached to imagine in detail their performance in an event. Research shows that athletes who do this type of vivid imagining actually experience small muscle contractions that reflect the bigger muscle movements they make in an actual performance.

Research has also documented the impact that thoughts, beliefs and attitudes have on our health. For example, there is evidence that a person's attitude after receiving a diagnosis of cancer can affect how long she or he lives. Simply stated, people who believe that a diagnosis of cancer is a death sentence do not survive as long as those who view the illness differently. Although many factors affect longevity in cancer patients, it appears that thoughts and beliefs can play a significant role.

LINDA: *The thought/physical reaction connection.*

When Linda's heart rate accelerated, she thought she was having a heart attack (Figure 2.1). This terrifying thought triggered a series of bodily changes, including quick, shallow breathing and profuse sweating. As Linda's breathing became more shallow, less oxygen was supplied to her heart, which caused her heart to beat even faster. Less oxygen was supplied to her brain, causing a sensation of dizziness and light-headedness.

PHYSICAL REACTIONS   **THOUGHTS**

Increased heart rate ——————→ I'm having a heart attack

More shallow breathing ↙

Less oxygen to heart and brain

Increased heart rate ——————→ This means I really am having
a heart attack. I'm going to die

Further increase in ↙
physical sensations

PANIC

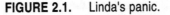

FIGURE 2.1.   Linda's panic.

Linda interpreted her increased heart rate and light-headedness as further signs of a heart attack. Following these thoughts, the physical sensations intensified. Her initial and subsequent thoughts that she was having a heart attack signaled immediate catastrophic danger. Her physical response to the perception of danger intensified until Linda experienced a panic attack. After a period of time in which she did not actually have a heart attack, Linda realized that she was panicking but not in danger, and her heart rate and breathing gradually slowed to normal.

WHAT IS THE THOUGHT/ENVIRONMENT CONNECTION?

Environment ─── (Thoughts)

At the beginning of this chapter you learned how thoughts influenced the moods we experience. You may be wondering why some people are more prone to certain thoughts and moods rather than others. Some portion of these differences may be biological or genetically inherited. But we also know that environmental experiences can powerfully shape the beliefs and moods that color our lives.

Recall that Marissa was sexually and physically abused throughout her childhood and early adult years. These experiences shaped her beliefs that she was worthless, unacceptable, and unlovable and that men were dangerous, abusive, and uncaring. It is understandable that Marissa's earliest attempts to make sense of her experiences led her to devalue herself and be on the lookout for the negative reactions of others.

It doesn't take traumatic environmental events to influence beliefs. Beliefs can be influenced by your cultural/ethnic background, gender, neighborhood, family beliefs and practices, religion, and the media. What you think about yourself, your future, and your life experiences is influenced by these parts of your early and current environment.

As an example of how culture influences beliefs, consider two children growing up. In many cultures, a girl would conclude from her environment that being pretty is the key to being well-liked. A boy would conclude that he should be strong and athletic to be well-liked.

There is nothing inherently more likable about beauty or strength, but our culture teaches us to make these connections. Once these beliefs are formed, they can be difficult to change. Therefore, many girls who are athletic find it difficult to value their skills, and boys with musical or artistic talents may feel cursed rather than blessed.

Vic was raised in a suburban community of educated professionals who valued achievement for themselves and their children. His family and school reflected these community values, emphasizing achievement and excellence. When Vic's performance in school or on the football field was not superior, his family, teachers, and friends were disappointed and reacted as if Vic had failed.

Based on these community reactions, Vic concluded that he was inadequate even though his performance was generally very good. Since Vic believed he was inadequate, it is not surprising that he felt anxious in situations that required him to perform and viewed football games and other performance situations as dangerous and a threat to his social standing because they entailed a risk of failure.

As you can see, Vic's childhood was not as traumatic as Marissa's. However, his childhood environment had equally as powerful an impact on the attitudes he developed and the thought patterns that persisted into adulthood.

EXERCISE: The Thought Connection

Worksheet 2.1 provides practice in recognizing the connection between thoughts and mood, behavior, and physical reactions.

WORKSHEET 2.1: The Thought Connection

Sarah, a 34-year-old woman, sat in the back row of the auditorium during a PTA meeting. She had concerns and questions regarding how her 8-year-old son was being taught and questions about classroom security. As Sarah was about to raise her hand to voice her concerns and questions she thought, "What if other people think my questions are stupid? Maybe I shouldn't ask these questions in front of the whole group. Someone may disagree with me and this could lead to a public argument. I could be humiliated."

Thought/Mood Connection
Based on Sarah's thoughts, which of the following moods is she likely to experience? (Check all that apply.)

_____ 1. Anxiety/Nervousness

_____ 2. Sadness

_____ 3. Happiness

_____ 4. Anger

_____ 5. Enthusiasm

Thought/Behavior Connection

Based on Sarah's thoughts, how do you predict she will behave?

_____ **1.** She will speak loudly and voice her concerns.

_____ **2.** She will remain silent.

_____ **3.** She will openly disagree with what other people say.

Thought/Physical Reaction Connection

Based on Sarah's thoughts, which of the following physical changes might she notice? (Check all that apply.)

_____ **1.** Rapid heart rate

_____ **2.** Sweaty palms

_____ **3.** Breathing changes

_____ **4.** Dizziness

When Sarah had these thoughts she felt anxious and nervous, remained silent, and experienced a rapid heart rate, sweaty palms, breathing changes, and dizziness. Were these the reactions you anticipated Sarah would have? Not everyone experiences the same reactions to particular thoughts. However, it is important to recognize that thoughts have mood, behavioral, and physical consequences.

IS POSITIVE THINKING THE SOLUTION?

Although our thoughts influence mood, behavior and physical reactions, positive thinking is not a solution to life's problems. Most people who are anxious, depressed or angry can tell you that "just thinking positive thoughts" is not that simple. In fact, if we do try to think only positive thoughts when we have a strong mood, we may miss important signals that something is wrong.

Cognitive therapy suggests instead that people consider as many different angles on a problem as possible. Looking at the situation from many different sides—positive and negative and neutral—can lead to new conclusions and solutions.

Suppose Marissa lost her job (remember, she had received written notices from her supervisor that her work was late or poorly done). If Marissa decided that she was fired because she was stupid and made too many mistakes and focused only on these ideas—she would probably have felt depressed and convinced that she could not be successful in any job.

However, if in addition to reviewing her mistakes, Marissa thought about her professional strengths, she could have focused more clearly on her strong skills and those that needed improvement as she looked for a new job. Marissa also could have considered alternative explanations for losing her job. Perhaps the job loss was not entirely or even at all her fault . Perhaps she was fired because of economic problems in the company or job discrimination.

You might wonder, "What difference does it make? Her job was gone!" Actually, it makes a big difference. If Marissa believed that the job loss was totally her fault, then the only solution was to change herself. If the job loss was even partly due to something else, then her responses and the solutions she considered might have been quite different: she might have felt angry and appealed the decision; she might have looked for a similar job in a more successful company.

IS CHANGING THE WAY YOU THINK THE ONLY WAY TO FEEL BETTER?

Even though identifying and changing thoughts is a central part of cognitive therapy, it is often equally important to make physical, behavioral, or environmental changes. For example, if you have been anxious for a long time, you probably avoid things that make you anxious. Part of dealing with anxiety is learning to relax (physical change) and to cope with perceived dangers so that you stop avoiding (behavioral change). People do not usually overcome anxiety until changes in thoughts are accompanied by changes in avoidance behavior.

To help you feel better, it also can be helpful to make changes in your environment. Reducing stress, learning to say no to unreasonable demands made by other people, spending more time with supportive people, working with neighbors to increase neighborhood safety, and using employee protections to reduce discrimination or harassment on the job are all environmental changes that can help you feel better.

Some environments are so challenging that it's difficult for anyone to maintain a positive outlook. For example, someone who is being abused by a family member probably needs help to either change or leave the situation. Just changing thoughts is not an adequate solution for abuse: The goal is to stop the abuse. Thought changes might help someone in this situation feel motivated to get help, but simply changing your thoughts to permit acceptance of the abuse is not the best solution.

As you complete the worksheets in this book, you will learn how to identify and change your thoughts, moods, behaviors, physical responses, and environment.

CHAPTER 2 SUMMARY

- Thoughts help define the moods we experience.

- Thoughts influence how we behave, what we choose to do and not do, and the quality of our performance.

- Thoughts and beliefs affect our biological responses.

- Environmental influences help determine the attitudes, beliefs, and thoughts that develop in childhood and often persist into adulthood.

- Cognitive therapy can help you look at all the information available; it is not simply positive thinking.

- While changes in thinking are often central, many problems require changes in behavior, physical functioning and environment, as well.

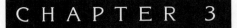

CHAPTER 3

Identifying and Rating Moods

In order to learn to manage or change your moods, it is helpful to be able to identify the moods you are experiencing. Moods can be difficult to identify. You may feel tired all the time and not recognize you are depressed. Or you might feel nervous and out of control and not recognize that you are anxious. Along with depression and anxiety, anger, shame, and guilt are very common moods that are problematic for people (see Chapters 10–12).

IDENTIFYING MOODS

The list below shows a variety of moods you might have during a day. This is not a comprehensive list: You can write additional moods on the blank lines. This list helps you pin down your moods more specifically than simply "bad" or "good." Notice that moods are usually described by one word. By identifying specific moods, you will be able to set goals for emotional change and track your progress toward those goals. Learning to distinguish between moods will enable you to choose actions designed to alleviate particular moods. For example, certain breathing techniques help nervousness but not depression.

26

MOOD LIST

Depressed	Anxious	Angry	Guilty	Ashamed
Sad	Embarrassed	Excited	Frightened	Irritated
Insecure	Proud	Mad	Panicky	Frustrated
Nervous	Disgusted	Hurt	Cheerful	Disappointed
Enraged	Scared	Happy	Loving	Humiliated
Other moods:	_____	_____	_____	_____

If you have trouble identifying your moods, notice changes in your body tension. Tight shoulders may signal that you are afraid or tense; a heaviness throughout your body may signal depression or disappointment.

A second way of becoming better at identifying your moods is to see if you can notice three different moods a day. If this is difficult to do, you may want to pick six of the moods from the list above and write down situations in your past in which you felt each one.

When Vic first began cognitive therapy, he thought he was feeling anxious and depressed. As he learned to identify moods, he discovered that he was also frequently angry. Although he had not had a drink for three years, he reported that he felt the urge to drink whenever he feared he would get "out of control." When he and his therapist looked closely at the times Vic sensed being "out of control," it became apparent that at these times he was feeling very nervous or angry. When nervous, Vic experienced a rapid heartbeat, sweaty hands, and a sense that something terrible was going to happen. He labeled these sensations being "out of control" and would have the urge to drink because he thought alcohol would help him regain control.

Vic obviously tended not to be very specific about his mood, often saying that he was "uncomfortable" or "numb." One of Vic's initial therapeutic tasks, therefore, was to begin to distinguish among his thoughts, moods, and behaviors in different situations in his life. In order to make the changes he wanted to make, Vic needed to be able to recognize the differences between these important parts of his experiences.

When Vic learned that his primary emotional difficulties were with anger and anxiety, he began to focus his attention on the situations in which he felt angry or anxious. He learned to distinguish his irritable anger from the fearful worry of his anxiety. He began to identify these moods, instead of lumping them together as "numbness." As Vic began to isolate what he was feeling, it became apparent to him that when his *mood* was anxious he was *thinking* "I'm losing control." When his *mood* was angry, he was *thinking*, "This is not fair—I deserve more respect."

Ben, at the beginning of therapy, said he did not feel like being with his family or friends as much as he used to. He said he preferred to be alone. As Ben began to closely analyze the situations from which he wanted to isolate himself, he discovered that he would often be *thinking* that others (family or friends) did not need him or want to be with him. He also realized that he was predicting (thinking) that if he got together with other people he would not have a good time. As he was *thinking* "They don't want to be with me" and "If I go there I'm not going to enjoy myself," he recognized that his mood was sad. During therapy, Ben learned the connection between his thoughts and moods and how to distinguish between them.

It was important for Vic and Ben to distinguish among situational factors (part of environment), thoughts, and moods. Situational factors can often be identified by answering the following questions:

1. Who was I with?

2. What was I doing?

3. When did it happen?

4. Where was I?

As a general rule, moods can be identified in one descriptive word. If it takes you more than one word to describe a mood, you may be describing a thought. Thoughts are the words or the visual images, including memories, that go through your mind.

The distinction among thoughts, moods, and situational factors is important for you to learn. By distinguishing among thoughts, moods, and situational factors, you can identify the parts of your experience that are in need of change.

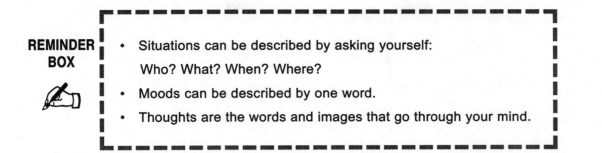

- Situations can be described by asking yourself:

  Who? What? When? Where?

- Moods can be described by one word.

- Thoughts are the words and images that go through your mind.

EXERCISE: Identifying Moods

Worksheet 3.1 is designed to help you identify your moods and set them apart from other important aspects of your life. In order to complete the worksheet, you need to focus on a specific situation in which you had an intense or powerful mood.

WORKSHEET 3.1: Identifying Moods

Describe a recent situation in which you had a strong mood. Next, identify what moods you had during or immediately after being in that situation. Do this for five different situations.

1. Situation: _____

    Moods: _____

2. Situation: _____

    Moods: _____

3. Situation: _____

    Moods: _____

4. Situation: _____

    Moods _____

5. Situation: _____

    Moods: _____

One of Vic's responses on Worksheet 3.1 looked like this:

SITUATION: *I'm alone, driving in my car, on the way to work at 7:45 A.M.*

MOODS: *Frightened, anxious, insecure*

One of Ben's responses was the following:

SITUATION: *I received a phone call from Max asking me to play golf.*

MOODS: *Sadness, grief*

As the examples illustrate, knowing the situation does not always help us understand why someone felt a particular emotion. Why would a golf invitation make Ben feel sad? The presence of strong moods is our first clue that something important is going on. Later chapters teach you why Ben and Vic—and you—experienced the particular moods described on Worksheet 3.1.

RATING MOODS

In addition to identifying moods, it is important to learn to rate the intensity of the moods you experience. Rating the intensity of the mood allows you to observe how your moods fluctuate. Rating your moods also helps alert you to which situations or thoughts are associated with changes in moods. Finally, you can use changes in emotional intensity to evaluate the effectiveness of strategies you are learning.

In order to see how your moods vary during the day, you'll find it convenient to use a rating scale. Ben and his therapist developed the following rating scale for his moods:

0	10	20	30	40	50	60	70	80	90	100
Not at all		A little			Medium		A lot		Most I've ever felt	

The therapist then asked Ben to use the scale to rate the moods he listed on Worksheet 3.1. For the golf invitation, Ben's ratings looked like this:

SITUATION: *I received a phone call from Max asking me to play golf.*

MOODS: *Sadness, grief*

Sadness	0	10	20	30	40	50	60	70	80	90	100
						X					

Grief	0	10	20	30	40	50	60	70	80	90	100
										X	

These ratings indicate that Ben experienced a high level of grief (90) and a medium level of sadness (50) while on the phone with Max.

EXERCISE: Rating Moods

On Worksheet 3.2, practice rating the intensity of your moods. On the blank lines, copy the situation and moods you identified on Worksheet 3.1. For each situation, rate one of the moods you identified on the scales provided. Circle the one mood you rated.

WORKSHEET 3.2: Identifying and Rating Moods

1. Situation: _____

Moods: _____

0	10	20	30	40	50	60	70	80	90	100

2. Situation: _____

Moods: _____

0	10	20	30	40	50	60	70	80	90	100

3. Situation: _____

Moods: _____

0	10	20	30	40	50	60	70	80	90	100

4. Situation: _____

Moods: _____

0   10   20   30   40   50   60   70   80   90   100
‾‾‾

5. Situation: _____

Moods: _____

0   10   20   30   40   50   60   70   80   90   100
‾‾‾

Since identifying and rating moods are important skills, continue to use Worksheet 3.2 to practice them until you can label and rate your moods easily. You may also want to read Chapters 10–12, which provide detailed descriptions of depression, anxiety, anger, guilt, and shame. The more you learn about moods, the easier it becomes to notice and name them. Once you are comfortable with identifying and rating moods, you are ready to proceed to Chapter 4.

CHAPTER 3 SUMMARY

- Strong moods signal that something important is going on in your life.

- Moods can usually be described in one word.

- Identifying specific moods can help you set and track goals, as well as enable you to choose interventions designed to alleviate particular moods.

- It is important to distinguish among situations, moods, and thoughts (Worksheet 3.2).

- Rating your moods (Worksheet 3.2) allows you to evaluate the strength and track the fluctuations of your emotional reactions.

CHAPTER 4

Situations, Moods, and Thoughts

One warm spring day in central California, a tennis coach was instructing a student on the art of serving the ball. While the student tossed and hit the ball over and over again, the coach focused attention on each part of the student's motion and swing. The coach never criticized the student, but instead gave feedback after each hit about the position of the racquet, the height of the ball toss, the angle of the racquet as it hit the ball, and the student's motion during the racquet follow-through.

In tennis, the ball needs to land in a service square in order to be a successful hit. Yet remarkably, the coach never once looked to see where the ball landed after the student hit it. Instead, the coach focused his feedback exclusively on suggestions for improving each part of the student's service stroke. The coach was confident that once the student learned each of the component skills, the student would be able to combine them so that the ball would consistently land in the proper area.

Just as this coach focused on development of specific skills, music teachers help students become better musicians by teaching notes, rhythms, and performance methods. Skilled laborers instruct their apprentices by showing them how to accomplish individual tasks on a work project. Each of these examples involves teaching *specific skills* and encouraging the learner to *practice* until these skills become familiar and easy to perform. We have all had experience with developing skills through practice (e.g., driving a car, diapering a baby, cooking a meal).

Fortunately, there is a set of specific skills that can help you learn to

THOUGHT

1. Situation	2. Moods	3. Automatic Thoughts (Images)
Who? What? When? Where?	**a.** What did you feel? **b.** Rate each mood (0–100%).	**a.** What was going though your mind just before you started to feel this way? Any other thoughts? Images? **b.** Circle the hot thought.

FIGURE 4.1. Sample Thought Record.

improve your mood, create desired behavior change, and change the thoughts that interfere with relationships. These skills are summarized on a 7-column worksheet called a "Thought Record" (Figure 4.1). Like the student practicing a tennis stroke, you will use parts of Thought Records many times in the weeks ahead to master the skills necessary to complete the whole worksheet.

RECORD

4. Evidence That Supports the Hot Thought	5. Evidence That Does Not Support the Hot Thought	6. Alternative/ Balanced Thoughts **a.** Write an alternative or balanced thought. **b.** Rate how much you believe in each alternative or balanced thought (0–100%).	7. Rate Moods Now Rerate moods listed in column 2 as well as any new moods (0–100%).

When Marissa's therapist first showed her a Thought Record, Marissa felt overwhelmed and depressed. The therapist used this reaction to help Marissa complete her first Thought Record (Figure 4.2). Notice that the first two columns of Marissa's Thought Record describe the situation she was in and what she was feeling, as you learned to do in Chapter 3. As her therapist helped Marissa fill out column 3, labeled "Automatic Thoughts (Images)" they uncovered certain thoughts that accompanied her emotional reactions. You will learn to uncover your own automatic thoughts and images in Chapter 5.

THOUGHT

1. Situation	2. Moods	3. Automatic Thoughts (Images)
Who? What? When? Where?	a. What did you feel? b. Rate each mood (0–100%).	a. What was going though your mind just before you started to feel this way? Any other thoughts? Images? b. Circle the hot thought.
Tues. 9:30 A.M. *In my therapist's office looking at the Thought Record*	*Overwhelmed 95%* *Depressed 85%*	*(This is too complicated for me to learn.)* *I'll never understand this.* *Image/memory: Taking a report card home with bad grades and being yelled at by my parents.* *I'll never get better.* *Nothing can help me.* *This therapy won't work.* *I'm doomed to always be depressed.*

FIGURE 4.2. Marissa's first Thought Record.

Marissa and her therapist next circled the thought ("This is too complicated for me to learn") that was strongly connected to her feeling overwhelmed. They wrote down evidence in columns 4 and 5 which did and did not support this thought. In column 6, they constructed alternative ways of looking at the situation based on the evidence in columns 4 and 5. They rated Marissa's belief in these alternative views 90%, 60% and 70%. As you see in column 7, completing this Thought Record lowered Marissa's feeling of being overwhelmed from 95% to 40% and her depression from 85% to 80%.

RECORD

4. Evidence That Supports the Hot Thought	5. Evidence That Does Not Support the Hot Thought	6. Alternative/ Balanced Thoughts a. Write an alternative or balanced thought. b. Rate how much you believe in each alternative or balanced thought (0–100%).	7. Rate Moods Now Rerate moods listed in column 2 as well as any new moods (0–100%).
I look at this thought record and I don't know what to do. I never was very good in school. I don't know what you mean by "evidence."	At work, I learned the computer filing system, which is complicated. Some of the early worksheets seemed hard until my therapist helped me do them a few times—then they seemed easier. My therapist said I need to know how to do only the first two columns now. I can get help from my therapist until I know how to do it on my own.	Even though this seems complicated now, I've learned other complicated things in the past. 90% My therapist will help show me how to do this. 60% With practice it might make sense and get easier. 70%	Over-whelmed 40% Depressed 80%

Chapter 6 shows you how to look for evidence for your automatic thoughts. In Chapter 7 you will learn how to use the evidence to construct more adaptive ways of thinking and viewing your life. The remainder of this chapter focuses on filling out columns 1–3 of the Thought Record using skills you have already learned.

COLUMN 1: Situation.

In Chapter 3, you learned to describe situations by answering questions. In filling out column 1 of the Thought Record, be as specific as possible. Describe the situation around you. Limit the "Situation" section to a specific time frame that does not exceed 30 minutes. For example, "all day Tuesday" is not workable. There are too many different situations, moods, and thoughts that can occur "all day Tuesday" to describe on the Thought Record. Marissa's description of her situation as "Tuesday, 9:30 A.M. in my therapist's office looking at the Thought Record" is a good example of a specific situation.

COLUMN 2: Moods.

In the "Moods" column of a Thought Record, list the moods you were experiencing in the situation you described. In addition to listing the moods, rate their intensity on a 0–100 scale.

Generally, moods can be described in one word. As you learned in Chapter 3, you can experience more than one mood in any situation. Each mood that you had in the situation you are recording should be listed and rated on the 0–100 scale. If you have trouble identifying the mood you were experiencing, you can refer to the Mood List on page 27 for help. If you describe your mood in an entire sentence, what you wrote may be a thought instead of a mood. If so, write the sentence in the "Thoughts" column and keep looking for a word to describe your mood in column 2.

People who experience panic attacks or anxiety may also want to record and rate the physical symptoms they experience along with their panic or anxiety (see Chapter 11). Since there is not a separate column for these symptoms, they can be recorded in the Mood column of the Thought Record. Physical symptoms can generally be described in one or two words (e.g., "heart racing 85%").

COLUMN 3: Thoughts.

In the "Automatic Thoughts (Images)" column, identify anything that went through your mind in the situation you described. Only those thoughts actually present in that situation should be recorded. Thoughts can be either verbal or visual. If they are images or memories, describe them in words. Notice that Marissa describes one of her thoughts as an image of bringing home a bad report card (Figure 4.2). Chapter 5 provides more detailed information to help you become proficient at identifying your thoughts.

As an example, Marissa brought the Thought Record in Figure 4.3 to her next therapy session. with the first three columns complete.

1. Situation	2. Moods	3. Automatic Thoughts (Images)
Who? What? When? Where?	**a.** What did you feel? **b.** Rate each mood (0–100%).	**a.** What was going though your mind just before you started to feel this way? Any other thoughts? Images? **b.** Circle the hot thought.
Wednesday, 2:45 P.M. My manager is coming to check on the progress I am making on the payroll project.	Depressed 90% Nervous 95% Afraid 97%	The project is not complete. What is complete is not OK. I'm failing. ⟨I'm going to be fired.⟩ It will be humiliating to have to tell my family that I've lost my job.

FIGURE 4.3.   Marissa's second Thought Record.

A second example shows how Vic reacted to an argument with his wife (Figure 4.4).

1. Situation	2. Moods	3. Automatic Thoughts (Images)
Who? What? When? Where?	**a.** What did you feel? **b.** Rate each mood (0–100%).	**a.** What was going though your mind just before you started to feel this way? Any other thoughts? Images? **b.** Circle the hot thought.
Friday, 6:00 P.M. Judy and I were arguing over which movie to go to.	Anger 99% Hurt 95% Sad 70%	She never cares about what I want to do. We always do what she wants to do. She always has to be in control. I would rather be numb and vegetate than feel this mad and hurt. I hate being angry all the time. I need a drink.

FIGURE 4.4. Vic's Thought Record.

Linda's Thought Record describing one of her first panic attacks is shown in Figure 4.5.

1. Situation	2. Moods	3. Automatic Thoughts (Images)
Who? What? When? Where?	a. What did you feel? b. Rate each mood (0–100%).	a. What was going though your mind just before you started to feel this way? Any other thoughts? Images? b. Circle the hot thought.
It is 2:30 in the afternoon. I'm alone at the mall, where I've been shopping for about 45 minutes.	Fear 100% Panic 100%	My heart is beginning to race. I'm starting to sweat. I may stop breathing. I can't get enough air. I'm dizzy. My chest feels tight. I'm having a heart attack. I'm losing control. (I'm going to die.) I need to get to a hospital. Image: I see myself lying on the floor, unable to breathe.

FIGURE 4.5. Linda's Thought Record.

Ben brought the Thought Record in Figure 4.6 to his therapist soon after beginning treatment.

1. Situation	2. Moods	3. Automatic Thoughts (Images)
Who? What? When? Where?	**a.** What did you feel? **b.** Rate each mood (0–100%).	**a.** What was going though your mind just before you started to feel this way? Any other thoughts? Images? **b.** Circle the hot thought.
Nov. 25. I'm preparing to go to Thanksgiving dinner at my daughter's home at 11:00 A.M.	*Sad 85%* *Remorseful 80%*	*Thanksgiving is such a sad time.* *I have two grown children who live out of town with their families.* *I don't get to see them nearly as often as I would like.* *Thanksgiving is the beginning of the season when families should be complete and together.* *We will never be a family like that again.* *(My life will never be as good as it once was.)*

FIGURE 4.6. Ben's Thought Record.

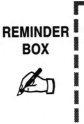

REMINDER BOX

- The "Situation" column of Thought Records focuses exclusively on Who? What? When? Where?

- Moods are identified in one word and rated for intensity on a 0-100 scale.

- The "Automatic Thoughts (Images)" column describes thoughts, beliefs, concerns, images, and meanings attached to the situations.

EXERCISE: Distinguishing Situations, Moods, and Thoughts

Worksheet 4.1 is an exercise to help you better distinguish your thoughts, moods, and situations. Write on the line at the right whether the item in the left column is a thought, mood, or situation. The first three items have been completed as examples.

WORKSHEET 4.1: Distinguishing Situations, Moods, and Thoughts

Situation, Mood, or Thought?

1. Nervous.   *mood*

2. At home.   *situation*

3. I'm not going to be able to do this.   *thought*

4. Sad. _____

5. Talking to a friend on the phone. _____

6. Irritated. _____

7. Driving in my car. _____

8. I'm always going to feel this way. _____

9. At work. _____

10. I'm going crazy. _____

11. Angry. _____

12. I'm no good. _____

13. 4:00 P.M. _____

14. Something terrible is going to happen. _____

15. Nothing ever goes right. _____

16. Discouraged _____

17. I'll never get over this. _____

18. Sitting in a restaurant. _____

19. I'm out-of-control. _____

20. I'm a failure. _____

21. Talking on the phone to my mom. _____

22. She's being inconsiderate. _____

23. Depressed. _____

24. I'm a loser. _____

25. Guilty. _____

26. At my son's house. _____

27. I'm having a heart attack. _____

28. I've been taken advantage of. _____

29. Lying in bed trying to go to sleep. _____

30. This isn't going to work out. _____

31. Shame. _____

32. I'm going to lose everything I've got. _____

33. Panic. _____

Following are answers to Worksheet 4.1. Review the pertinent sections of this chapter to clarify any differences between your answers and the ones given.

1. Nervous. ....Mood
2. At home. ....Situation
3. I'm not going to be able to do this. ....Thought
4. Sad. ....Mood
5. Talking to a friend on the phone. ....Situation
6. Irritated. ....Mood
7. Driving in my car. ....Situation
8. I'm always going to feel this way. ....Thought
9. At work. ....Situation
10. I'm going crazy. ....Thought
11. Angry. ....Mood
12. I'm no good. ....Thought
13. 4:00 P.M. ....Situation
14. Something terrible is going to happen. ....Thought
15. Nothing ever goes right. ....Thought
16. Discouraged. ....Mood
17. I'll never get over this. ....Thought

18. Sitting in a restaurant. ....Situation
19. I'm out-of-control. ....Thought
20. I'm a failure. ....Thought
21. Talking on the phone to my mom. ....Situation
22. She's being inconsiderate. ....Thought
23. Depressed. ....Mood
24. I'm a loser. ....Thought
25. Guilty. ....Mood
26. At my son's house. ....Situation
27. I'm having a heart attack. ....Thought
28. I've been taken advantage of. ....Thought
29. Lying in bed trying to go to sleep. .... Situation
30. This isn't going to work out. ....Thought
31. Shame. ....Mood
32. I'm going to lose everything I've got. ....Thought
33. Panic. ....Mood

If you had difficulty distinguishing among situations, moods, and thoughts, review Chapters 3 and 4. It is important to distinguish these parts of your experience in order to make changes in your life. By separating these components from each other, you will be better able to make changes that are important to you.

CHAPTER 4 SUMMARY

- Thought Records help develop a set of skills that can improve your mood and relationships and lead to positive behavior change.

- The first 3 columns of a Thought Record distinguish a situation from the feelings and thoughts you had in the situation.

- A Thought Record lists evidence that does and does not support thoughts you identified.

- Thought Records provide an opportunity to develop new ways of thinking that can lead to feeling better.

- As in developing any new skill, you will need to practice completing many thought records before consistent results are achieved.

CHAPTER 5

Automatic Thoughts

Marissa was working at her desk when her supervisor came in to say hello. While they were talking her supervisor said, "By the way, I want to compliment you on the nice report you wrote yesterday." As soon as her supervisor said this, Marissa became nervous and scared. She couldn't shake this mood the rest of the morning.

Vic was putting the dishes on the counter after dinner when his wife said, "I took the car in to get the oil changed today." With irritation, Vic said, "I told you I was going to change the oil on Saturday." His wife replied, "Well, you've been saying you'd take care of it for two weeks, so I just took care of it myself." "Fine!" yelled Vic, throwing a dish towel across the room. "Why don't you just get yourself another husband!" He grabbed his coat and slammed the door as he left the house.

As you begin keeping track of your moods, you will notice times when you, like Marissa, experience a mood that doesn't seem to fit the situation. Most people don't feel anxious after getting a compliment. At other times, you will have a quick, strong reaction like Vic. An outsider looking on this scene might think Vic is reacting too much in this situation, yet this reaction might seem to be just the right one to him.

How can we make sense of our moods? By identifying the thoughts we are having, our moods usually make perfect sense. Think of thoughts as a clue to understanding mood. For Marissa, we have the following puzzle:

SITUATION	CLUE: THOUGHTS	MOOD
Receive a compliment from my supervisor	???	Nervous 80% Scared 90%

How can this make sense? Marissa was confused about why she reacted this way until she talked to her therapist.

THERAPIST: What was scary about this situation?

MARISSA: I don't know—just knowing the supervisor noticed my work, I guess.

THERAPIST: What's scary about that?

MARISSA: Well, I don't always do a good job.

THERAPIST: So what might happen?

MARISSA: Some day the supervisor will notice a mistake.

THERAPIST: And then what might happen?

MARISSA: The supervisor will be mad at me.

THERAPIST: What's the worst that might happen then?

MARISSA: I hadn't thought about it, but I - I guess I could get fired.

THERAPIST: And then what might happen?

MARISSA: With a bad recommendation, I'd have trouble getting another job.

THERAPIST: Can you summarize, Marissa, what your thoughts were that help explain why you were scared after receiving your supervisor's compliment?

MARISSA: Now I can see that the compliment made me realize my supervisor is noticing my work. Since I know I make mistakes, I thought about what might happen if my supervisor noticed one of these mistakes. I guess I jumped to the conclusion that I'd be fired and not be able to get another job. It sounds a little silly now.

Notice how the thoughts uncovered by Marissa and her therapist provide the necessary clues to understand her emotional reaction.

SITUATION	CLUE: THOUGHTS	MOOD
Receive a compliment from my supervisor	I'll make a mistake, be fired, and won't be able to get another job.	Nervous 80% Scared 90%

Most of us would feel nervous and scared if we thought we were going to be fired and couldn't get another job. Now Marissa's moods make sense. As you can see, an important step in understanding our moods is learning to identify the thoughts that accompany them.

See if you can guess what Vic's automatic thoughts might have been when he got so angry with his wife for changing the oil in the car.

SITUATION	CLUE: THOUGHTS	MOOD
Judy changed oil in car. Judy says, "You've been saying you'd take care of it for two weeks, so I just took care of it myself."		Angry 95%

In the "Clue: Thoughts" column, write any thoughts you can think of that would explain Vic's strong, angry reaction.

After Vic left the house, he realized that he was not upset that his wife had changed the oil in the car. In fact, his week had been very busy and it was a big help that she had taken care of this chore. His anger was related to the *thoughts* he had about her changing the oil. He thought, "She's mad at me for not doing it. She doesn't appreciate how hard I'm trying to do everything. She is critical of me, she thinks I'm not good enough. No matter how hard I try, she's never happy with me."

These thoughts help us understand Vic's reactions. Thoughts like these are called *automatic thoughts* because they simply pop into our heads automatically throughout the day. We don't plan or intend to think a certain way. In fact, we usually are not even aware of our automatic thoughts. One of the purposes of cognitive therapy is to bring automatic thoughts into awareness.

Awareness is the first step toward change and better problem solving. Once Vic was aware of his thoughts, a number of possibilities for change became available to him. If he decided that his thoughts were unreasonable or didn't work for him, he could work to alter his understanding of the situation. On the other hand, if Vic concluded that his thoughts were reasonable, he could talk directly to his wife to discuss his feelings and ask her to appreciate his efforts more.

HOW DO WE BECOME AWARE OF OUR OWN AUTOMATIC THOUGHTS?

Since we are constantly thinking and imagining, we have automatic thoughts all the time. We daydream about lunch or the weekend or worry about getting errands done. These are all automatic thoughts. The automatic thoughts that are of interest in this book are the ones that help us understand our strong moods. These thoughts can be *words* ("I'll be fired"), *images* or mental pictures (Marissa might have "seen" herself as a homeless person pushing a shopping cart down the street), or *memories* (the memory of being hit on the hand with a ruler by her fifth-grade teacher when she made a mistake might have flashed through Marissa's mind.)

HELPFUL HINTS

☞

To identify automatic thoughts, notice what goes through your mind when you have a strong feeling or a strong reaction to something.

To practice identifying automatic thoughts, write down what goes through your mind when you imagine yourself in the following situations.

1. **Situation:** You are at a shopping mall and are going to buy a very special present for yourself. You saw it there a few weeks ago and have been saving your money to buy it. When you get to the store, the sales clerk tells you they no longer carry that item.

   Automatic thoughts:_____

   _____

   _____

   _____

   _____

   _____

2. **Situation:** You cooked chili for a neighborhood party. You are a bit nervous because you tried a new recipe. After 10 minutes several people come up and say they think the chili is delicious.

   Automatic thoughts:_____

   _____

   _____

   _____

   _____

   _____

Different people have different automatic thoughts in these situations. For the chili situation in example 2, some people think, "Oh good, the chili turned out OK," and they feel relief or pride. Other people might think, "These people are just trying not to hurt my feelings; it probably tastes lousy," and they might feel ashamed or embarrassed. As you can see, in any situation there are many ways to interpret what the events mean. The interpretation you make determines your mood.

Actually, we usually have several automatic thoughts during real situations in our lives. The questions in the box can help you identify your automatic thoughts. Not every question will help you in every situation, but by asking yourself each of these questions you will increase the likelihood of capturing most of your automatic thoughts.

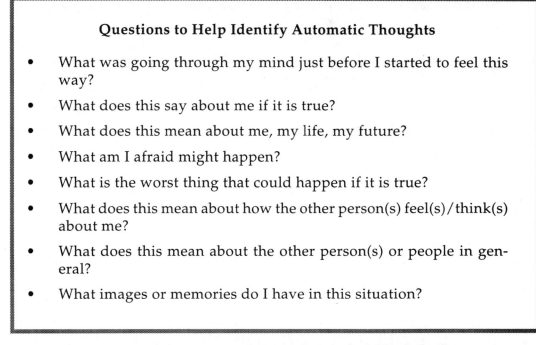

To identify automatic thoughts in situations, ask yourself these questions until you have identified the thoughts that help you understand your emotional reactions. You may need to ask yourself some of these questions two or three times to uncover all of the automatic thoughts. To look for images and memories, just let your mind wander and see if any pictures come to mind when you think of the situation where you had the strong feeling.

EXERCISE: Separating Situations, Moods, and Thoughts

Think of a time today or yesterday when you had a particularly strong feeling such as depression, anger, or anxiety. Write about this experience, on Worksheet 5.1 (on the following page), describing the situation, your moods, and your thoughts in as much detail as you can remember. This exercise is designed to help you define, separate, and understand the different parts of your experience, an important step in learning to be more in control of your moods.

WORKSHEET 5.1: Separating Situations, Moods, and Thoughts

1. Situation	2. Moods	3. Automatic Thoughts (Images)
		Answer some or all of the following questions: What was going through my mind just before I started to feel this way? What does this say about me? What does this mean about me? my life? my future? What am I afraid might happen? What is the worst thing that could happen if this is true? What does this mean about how the other person(s) feel(s)/think(s) about me? What does this mean about the other person(s) or people in general? What images or memories do I have in this situation?
Who were you with? What were you doing? When was it? Where were you?	Describe each mood in one word. Rate intensity of mood (0–100%).	

Learning to identify automatic thoughts can be very interesting, and identifying them will help you understand why you feel the way you feel in different situations. The more you pay attention to your thoughts, the easier it is to identify several thoughts tied to a mood.

EXERCISE: Identifying Automatic Thoughts

Worksheet 5.2 is designed to give you more practice in identifying your automatic thoughts. Automatic thoughts are the springboard for change throughout the remaining chapters of this book. Therefore, it is important for you to become adept at identifying them. Before reading ahead, complete Worksheet 5.2 (on the following page) for another situation in which you had a strong feeling. Use the questions at the bottom of column 3 (from box page 51) to help you identify what you are thinking. For this column you do not need to answer every question. Ask yourself whichever questions help you identify your automatic thoughts in this situation.

WORKSHEET 5.2: Identifying Automatic Thoughts

1. Situation	2. Moods	3. Automatic Thoughts (Images)
		Answer some or all of the following questions: What was going through my mind just before I started to feel this way? What does this say about me? What does this mean about me? my life? my future? What am I afraid might happen? What is the worst thing that could happen if this is true? What does this mean about how the other person(s) feel(s)/think(s) about me?
Who were you with? What were you doing? When was it? Where were you?	Describe each mood in one word. Rate intensity of mood (0–100%).	What does this mean about the other person(s) or people in general? What images or memories do I have in this situation?

From *Mind Over Mood* by Dennis Greenberger and Christine A. Padesky. © 1995 The Guilford Press.

Identifying your automatic thoughts is an important step in feeling better and coping better. Chapters 6, 7, 8, and 9 teach you what to do with these thoughts to help you feel better.

HOT THOUGHTS

Perhaps you have had the experience of walking into a room, turning on the lamp switch, and having no light appear. You may have discovered that the wall switch connected to the lamp's plug was turned off so the lamp was not receiving electricity. Activating the wall switch causes electricity to flow in the circuit, allowing the lamp to turn on.

Wires that carry electricity are called "hot" wires. Similarly, the automatic thoughts that are most connected to moods are called "hot" thoughts. These are the thoughts that conduct the emotional charge, so these are also the thoughts that are important for us to identify, examine, and sometimes alter to feel better.

To learn about hot automatic thoughts, let's look at one of Vic's Thought Records (Figure 5.1 on the following page). To help identify his automatic thoughts, Vic asked himself the questions in the box on page 51. These questions are underlined.

1. Situation	2. Moods	3. Automatic Thoughts (Images)
Who? What? When? Where?	a. What did you feel? b. Rate each mood (0–100%).	a. What was going though your mind just before you started to feel this way? Any other thoughts? Images? b. Circle the hot thought.
Handing a monthly report to my supervisor. She reads it standing in my office. Tuesday, 4:30 P.M.	Nervous 90% Irritated 60%	_What was going through my mind just before I got nervous?_ Why is she reading it here? _What am I afraid might happen?_ She'll be unhappy with my sales. I bet the others did better this month. _What does this say about me if it is true?_ This means I'm no good. _What might happen if this is true?_ I'll get fired or get a pay cut. _What went through my mind just before I got irritated?_ I never get credit for how hard I work. _What does this mean about other people?_ It means other people are always critical and I'll never get ahead—it's not fair. _What images or memories do I have in this situation?_ A memory of my dad criticizing how I mowed the lawn.

FIGURE 5.1: Vic's Thought Record.

Notice that Vic described the situation and then identified and rated his moods. To figure out the automatic thoughts connected with his nervousness, he asked himself some of the questions listed in the box on page 51.

After he identified a number of thoughts to help explain his nervous feeling, Vic then asked himself questions to help identify the automatic thoughts connected to his irritated feeling. Finally, Vic asked himself to look for images and memories and remembered a time when he felt the same way he did on this day.

To find out which of his thoughts were hottest—most emotionally charged—Vic considered each thought by itself to see how much that thought alone would make him feel either nervous or irritated. For example, if he thought only the first thought—"Why is she reading it here?"—Vic decided he would have rated his nervousness 10. However, when he thought "She'll be unhappy with my sales," his nervousness rating jumped to 40. All of Vic's ratings can be seen here:

THOUGHT	MOOD
Why is she reading it here?	Nervous 10%
She'll be unhappy with my sales.	Nervous 40%
I bet the others did better this month	Nervous 80%
This means I'm no good.	Nervous 90%
I'll get fired or get a paycut.	Nervous 90%
I never get credit for how hard I work.	Irritated 40%
Other people are always critical.	Irritated 40%
I'll never get ahead—it's not fair.	Irritated 80%
Memory of my dad criticizing how I mowed the lawn.	Irritated 60% Nervous 90%

As you can see, Vic's first thought was not strongly tied to mood, so it is not particularly hot. His next four thoughts were related to his mood of nervousness, so all four thoughts were hot thoughts. Three of the four ("I bet the others did better this month," "This means I'm no good," and "I'll get fired or get a pay cut") make Vic extremely nervous, and so these are the hottest thoughts. Which of Vic's thoughts are hot thoughts for his irritation? Which are the hottest thoughts? Looking for more automatic thoughts by asking yourself questions, as Vic did, makes it more likely that you will find hot thoughts to help you understand your emotional reactions.

There is one last thing of importance on Vic's Thought Record. Notice that the childhood memory he recalled was a hot thought for both irritation (60%) and nervousness (90%). This memory seemed closely tied to his reaction to the supervisor. Later, Vic learned to look for similarities and differences between the supervisor reading his report and his dad criticizing his lawn mowing. Being aware of this memory and learning to see the differences between his childhood experiences and his adult experiences will help Vic learn to react in more adaptive ways with both his supervisor and his wife.

EXERCISE: Identifying Hot Thoughts

Now you are ready to identify your own hot thoughts. For each of the automatic thoughts you listed on Worksheet 5.2, rate how much (0–100%) this thought alone made you feel the emotion you listed. Write the rating next to each thought. These ratings will help you decide which one(s) are the hot thoughts. Do these thoughts help you understand why you had the particular moods? For Worksheet 5.2, circle the hot thoughts for each mood. If none of the thoughts listed are hot, ask yourself the questions in the box on page 51 to try again to identify additional automatic thoughts.

The skills taught in this chapter are so important that the chapter ends with a special Thought Record. Worksheet 5.3 is similar to Worksheet 5.2, with the addition of a fourth column in which you can rate the hotness of each automatic thought you identify. Notice the helpful hints and questions at the bottom of column 3 which remind you what information to include in the "Automatic Thoughts" column.

Use Worksheet 5.3 until you can successfully identify your automatic thoughts and find the hot thoughts connected to your moods. We recommend that you complete Worksheet 5.3 at least once a day for one week. This skill is necessary in order to evaluate your thoughts and make changes if you determine that there is a more adaptive or healthier way of thinking.

The more Thought Records you do, the faster you will feel better. Doing a Thought Record is not a test. It is an exercise in identifying your thoughts and thought patterns that will build your skill in recognizing how your moods and thoughts influence your daily life. With continual practice, you will become more skilled in completing Thought Records. As your skill increases you are likely to feel better, less depressed, less anxious, happier and more in control of your life. Once you are skilled at doing columns 1–3 of a Thought Record, you are ready for the rest of this book.

WORKSHEET 5.3: Identifying Hot Thoughts

1. Situation	2. Moods	3. Automatic Thoughts (Images)	Rate Hotness of Each Thought
Who were you with? What were you doing? When was it? Where were you?	Describe each mood in one word. Rate intensity of mood (0–100%).	**Answer some or all of the following questions:** What was going through my mind just before I started to feel this way? What does this say about me? What does this mean about me? my life? my future? What am I afraid might happen? What is the worst thing that could happen if this is true? What does this mean about how the other person(s) feel(s)/think(s) about me? What does this mean about the other person(s) or people in general? Do I have any images or memories in this situation? If so, what are they?	For each thought in column 3, rate from 0 to100% how much emotion you would experience based on that thought alone.

WORKSHEET 5.3: Identifying Hot Thoughts

1. Situation	2. Moods	3. Automatic Thoughts (Images)	Rate Hotness of Each Thought
		Answer some or all of the following questions: What was going through my mind just before I started to feel this way? What does this say about me? What does this mean about me? my life? my future? What am I afraid might happen? What is the worst thing that could happen if this is true? What does this mean about how the other person(s) feel(s)/think(s) about me? What does this mean about the other person(s) or people in general? Do I have any images or memories in this situation? If so, what are they?	
Who were you with? What were you doing? When was it? Where were you?	Describe each mood in one word. Rate intensity of mood (0–100%).		For each thought in column 3, rate from 0 to100% how much emotion you would experience based on that thought alone.

From *Mind Over Mood* by Dennis Greenberger and Christine A. Padesky. © 1995 The Guilford Press.

WORKSHEET 5.3: Identifying Hot Thoughts

1. Situation	2. Moods	3. Automatic Thoughts (Images)	Rate Hotness of Each Thought
Who were you with? What were you doing? When was it? Where were you?	Describe each mood in one word. Rate intensity of mood (0–100%).	**Answer some or all of the following questions:** What was going through my mind just before I started to feel this way? What does this say about me? What does this mean about me? my life? my future? What am I afraid might happen? What is the worst thing that could happen if this is true? What does this mean about how the other person(s) feel(s)/think(s) about me? What does this mean about the other person(s) or people in general? Do I have any images or memories in this situation? If so, what are they?	For each thought in column 3, rate from 0 to 100% how much emotion you would experience based on that thought alone.

CHAPTER 5 SUMMARY

- Automatic thoughts are thoughts that come into our minds spontaneously throughout the day.

- Whenever we have strong moods, there are also automatic thoughts present that provide clues to understanding our emotional reactions.

- Automatic thoughts can be words, images, or memories.

- To identify automatic thoughts, notice what goes through your mind when you have a strong mood.

- Hot thoughts are automatic thoughts that carry the strongest emotional charge.

CHAPTER 6

Where's the Evidence?

VIC: *Stop, look, and relisten.*

One Thursday evening, Vic and his wife, Judy, were standing in the kitchen discussing their plans for the forthcoming weekend. Vic told Judy that he had made plans for Saturday morning to meet his friend Jim at an Alcoholics Anonymous (AA) meeting. Judy's expression changed as he spoke and a look of distress came over her face. Vic experienced a surge of anger as he thought, "She's upset I'm spending time away from her and the kids. It's not fair that she doesn't see my recovery program as important. If she cared about me as much as the kids, she'd be happy I was going. She doesn't care about me."

Vic exploded at Judy: "If you don't care about my sobriety, then I don't care either!" He slammed his fist on the table and stormed out of the house. As he left Judy yelled after him, "How can you expect me to care when you act like this? What's wrong with you?"

As Vic drove away from the house, his thoughts were racing. "She's never understood how important AA is to me. She doesn't know how hard it is not to drink. What's the use in trying so hard if she doesn't care if I stay sober? I can't stand being so angry. A drink will make me feel better."

As Vic neared the bar he used to stop at every night, he pulled his car into a parking lot and turned off the ignition. He put his head on the steering wheel to catch his breath. As his anger began to subside, he remembered his therapist telling him about three of the most important words in cognitive therapy. When he was feeling angry or anxious or had a strong impulse to drink, his therapist had told him to ask himself, "Where's the evidence?" Vic began to consider evidence to support his thoughts that Judy was upset with his plans to go to AA and that she didn't care or support his sobriety.

Vic's anger was based on interpreting the look on his wife's face as irritation with his decision to attend a Saturday AA meeting. By looking for evidence that did and did not support his conclusions, Vic put himself in a better position to evaluate and react to what was going on between him and

THOUGHT

1. Situation	2. Moods	3. Automatic Thoughts (Images)
Who? What? When? Where?	a. What did you feel? b. Rate each mood (0–100%)	a. What was going though your mind just before you started to feel this way? Any other thoughts? Images? b. Circle the hot thought
Thursday, 8:30 P.M. Judy gives me an odd look when I tell her I'm going to AA on Saturday	Anger 90%	She's upset that I'm going to AA on Saturday. She doesn't see my recovery program as important. (She doesn't care about me.) She doesn't understand how hard it is not to drink. I can't stand being so angry. A drink will make me feel better.

FIGURE 6.1. Vic's Thought Record.

Judy. He also gathered more information that could assist him in controlling his anger and his drinking.

Columns 4 and 5 of the Thought Record address the question "Where's the evidence?" (Figure 6.1). These two columns are designed to help you gather information that supports and does not support the hot thoughts you identified in the "Automatic Thoughts" column. The information collected in columns 4 and 5 can provide a basis for evaluating your hot thoughts.

When you begin filling out the two evidence columns, it is helpful to consider your hot thoughts as hypotheses, or guesses. If you temporarily suspend your conviction that your hot thoughts are true, you will find it easier to look for evidence that both supports and weakens your conclusion.

As Vic sat in his car outside the bar considering the evidence for and against conclusions about the situation with Judy, he rummaged through papers in his briefcase for a Thought Record, which he filled out out as you see in Figure 6.1.

RECORD

4. Evidence That Supports the Hot Thought	5. Evidence That Does Not Support the Hot Thought	6. Alternative/ Balanced Thoughts a. Write an alternative or balanced thought. b. Rate how much you believe in each alternative or balanced thought (0–100%).	7. Rate Moods Now Rerate moods listed in column 2 as well as any new moods. (0–100%).
She's not supportive of AA. She nags me to do things. She doesn't seem to appreciate how hard I work. She's always giving me negative looks like tonight. She yelled at me as I was leaving the house.	She stuck with me during all those years of drinking. She attended Al-Anon meetings for a year. She seemed happy to see me when I came home from work tonight. She tells me she loves me and does nice things for me when we're not fighting.		

As you learned to do in Chapter 5, Vic filled out the first three columns of the Thought Record by describing the situation, identifying and rating his mood, and writing down a variety of thoughts connected to his mood. Instead of writing out his ratings of how "hot" each automatic thought was, Vic mentally considered how angry each thought made him feel and circled the hottest thought, "She doesn't care about me."

In columns 4 and 5, Vic drew on his experiences with Judy to list details that supported or did not support this hot thought. He considered data, facts, or experiences that did or did not support his hot thought rather than his opinions.

The information in the evidence columns of a Thought Record should consist mostly of objective data or facts. However, when you first begin to fill out these columns, you will probably mix facts with interpretations, as Vic did on his Thought Record. For example, Vic wrote, "She's always giving me negative looks like tonight," which reflects his interpretation that her distressed look was a negative look directed at him. This statement may be an exaggeration of how often Judy gives him negative looks.

As you practice completing the evidence columns for your own automatic thoughts, try to be objective in the data you write. However, even if you do include some data which are not objective in column 4, the Thought Record will be valuable if you can find evidence to write in column 5. This column is one of the most important on the Thought Record because it asks you to look for information that contradicts your conclusions. *Evidence showing that our beliefs are not completely true can be hard to uncover when we are experiencing a strong mood. Yet, looking at the evidence both for and against our conclusions is the secret to reducing the intensity of the mood.*

BEN: *Second thoughts.*

An example from Ben's life further illustrates the importance of relying on evidence to evaluate conclusions. Approximately four months after his therapy began, Ben felt very sad as he returned home from a day spent visiting his daughter and her family. After he arrived at home, Ben decided to write a Thought Record in order to better understand his sadness and as an attempt to feel better.

After identifying a series of automatic thoughts, Ben decided that they were all "hot." However, the ones that seemed most connected to his sadness were the ideas that he wasn't needed any more by his children and grandchildren and that no one paid attention to him that day. Ben circled these hottest thoughts on the Thought Record in Figure 6.2 on pages 68 and 69.

When we have negative automatic thoughts, we usually dwell on data that confirms our conclusions. Before writing out his Thought Record, Ben's thoughts were focused on the column 4 events which supported his belief that, "the kids and grandkids don't need me any more." Thinking only about the ways in which he was no longer needed by his family led Ben to feel very sad.

Column 5 of the Thought Record required Ben to actively search his memory for experiences that contradicted his conclusions. When Ben recalled events that indicated that he was still needed and loved by his family, his mood lifted. Even though his children were grown up and his grandchildren were doing more things for themselves, Ben was able to remember events suggesting that he was still an important person in their lives.

The realization of his importance to his family was not available to Ben as long as he focused only on evidence that his negative thoughts were true. Column 5 encouraged Ben to actively remember and examine information that was contradictory to his original negative automatic thoughts.

Like Ben, you will probably experience a shift in mood if you can find evidence to write in column 5. However, if you are experiencing a very strong mood or holding a belief that seems absolutely true to you, it can be hard to see the evidence that does not support your beliefs. The questions in the Hint Box on page 70, which remind you to look at a situation from many different perspectives, will help you find contradictory evidence.

THOUGHT

1. Situation	2. Moods	3. Automatic Thoughts (Images)
Who? What? When? Where?	a. What did you feel? b. Rate each mood (0–100%).	a. What was going though your mind just before you started to feel this way? Any other thoughts? Images? b. Circle the hot thought
November 25, 9:00 P.M. Driving home from my daughter's home where I spent Thanksgiving with my daughter, son-in-law, two of my grandchildren, and my wife.	Sad 80%	They all would have had a better time if I hadn't been there today. They didn't pay any attention to me all day. The kids and grandkids don't need me anymore.

FIGURE 6.2. Ben's Thought Record.

RECORD

4. Evidence That Supports the Hot Thought	5. Evidence That Does Not Support the Hot Thought	6. Alternative/ Balanced Thoughts a. Write an alternative or balanced thought. b. Rate how much you believe in each alternative or balanced thought (0–100%).	7. Rate Moods Now Rerate moods listed in column 2 as well as any new moods. (0–100%).
I used to enjoy tying my granddaughter's shoes, but now she wants to do this on her own. My daughter and son-in-law have their lives together and they don't need anything from me. Amy, the 15-year-old, left at 7:00 P.M. to be with her friends. Bill, my son-in-law, built new shelves and cabinets in the family room. Three years ago he would have asked me and needed me to help him with a project that big.	Bill asked for my advice on plans for a room addition to their home. My daughter asked me to take a look at some vegetables in their garden that were dying. I was able to tell her that they weren't getting enough water. I made my 5-year-old granddaughter laugh often throughout the day. Amy seemed to enjoy my stories about her mom as a teenager. My 5-year-old granddaughter fell asleep in my lap.		

**HELPFUL
HINTS**

☞

QUESTIONS TO HELP FIND EVIDENCE THAT DOES NOT SUPPORT YOUR HOT THOUGHT

- Have I had any experiences that show that this thought is not completely true all the time?

- If my best friend or someone I loved had this thought, what would I tell them?

- If my best friend or someone who loves me knew I was thinking this thought, what would they say to me? What evidence would they point out to me that would suggest that my thoughts were not 100% true?

- When I am not feeling this way, do I think about this type of situation any differently? How?

- When I have felt this way in the past, what did I think about that helped me feel better?

- Have I been in this type of situation before? What happened? Is there anything different between this situation and previous ones? What have I learned from prior experiences that could help me now?

- Are there any small things that contradict my thoughts that I might be discounting as not important?

- Five years from now, if I look back at this situation, will I look at it any differently? Will I focus on any different part of my experience?

- Are there any strengths or positives in me or the situation that I am ignoring?

- Am I jumping to any conclusions in columns 3 and 4 that are not completely justified by the evidence?

- Am I blaming myself for something over which I do not have complete control?

MARISSA: *Put yourself in someone else's . . . head.*

In the beginning of her therapy, Marissa encountered some difficulty in answering the question "Where's the evidence?" Marissa brought the partially completed Thought Record in Figure 6.3 (pages 72 and 73) to one of her early therapy sessions.

On her own, Marissa was unable to unearth any evidence that her hot thought was not 100% true. The following interchange with her therapist helped her access information important in completing column 5. Notice that the questions Marissa's therapist asked are similar to those in the Hint Box on page 70.

THERAPIST:	If I understand your Thought Record correctly, your hot thought was "The pain is so great that I have to kill myself." You were able to find evidence to support that thought, but you were unable to find any evidence that did not support this thought.
MARISSA:	That's right.
THERAPIST:	Have you ever felt in the past that your pain was so great that you had to kill yourself?
MARISSA:	Dozens of times.
THERAPIST:	In the past when you have felt this way, what have you done or thought about that has helped you to feel better?
MARISSA:	It's funny, but sometimes talking about my pain helps me feel better.
THERAPIST:	So talking about it helps. In the past have you ever thought about anything that has helped you to feel better?
MARISSA:	When I'm feeling the worst I try to remember that I have felt this way before and have gotten through it every time.
THERAPIST:	Well, that is important information. Is there anything about your situation now that suggests that suicide is not the only option?
MARISSA:	What do you mean?
THERAPIST:	I'm wondering whether or not you have any hope that something other than suicide will lessen your pain?
MARISSA:	Well, I guess I'm learning to think differently, but I'm not so sure that's going to help.
THERAPIST:	Part of you is doubtful about whether the cognitive therapy will help you and part of you is hopeful.
MARISSA:	I am much more doubtful than hopeful.
THERAPIST:	Percent-wise, how much of you is doubtful and how much of you is hopeful that the skills you are learning will help lessen your pain?

MARISSA:	I am 90 to 95% doubtful and 5 to 10% hopeful.
THERAPIST:	We'll keep track of how your levels of doubt and hopefulness fluctuate as you progress in therapy. If you told your best friend, Kate, that "The pain is so great that I have to kill myself" what would she say to you?
MARISSA:	I never would tell her, but if I did she probably would tell me that I have a lot going for me, a lot to look forward to, and a lot to contribute to the world. I wouldn't believe her, though.
THERAPIST:	Would she tell you anything else that you might partially believe?
MARISSA:	She would probably point out that there are some things in

THOUGHT

1. Situation	2. Moods	3. Automatic Thoughts (Images)
Who? What? When? Where?	**a.** What did you feel? **b.** Rate each mood (0–100%).	**a.** What was going though your mind just before you started to feel this way? Any other thoughts? Images? **b.** Circle the hot thought.
At home alone, Saturday, 9:30 P.M.	Depressed 100% Disappointed 95% Empty 100% Confused 90% Unreal 95%	I want to go numb so I don't have to feel anymore. I'm not making any progress. I'm so confused that I can't think clearly. I don't know what's real and what isn't. ⟨The pain is so great that I have to kill myself.⟩ Nothing helps. Life is not worth living. I'm such a failure.

FIGURE 6.3. Marissa's partially completed Thought Record.

life that give me some enjoyment, that I have some moments during most days when I feel better and in less pain. She would remind me that some things strike me as funny and I laugh occasionally.

THERAPIST: If Kate told you that she was experiencing severe emotional pain and thought that suicide was the only solution what would you say to her?

MARISSA: I would tell her to keep trying other solutions. There would have to be hope for Kate. But I don't see much hope for me.

THERAPIST: We'll consider how much hope makes sense in a few minutes. First, let's write on the Thought Record the things we just talked about that can go in column 5.

RECORD

4. Evidence That Supports the Hot Thought	5. Evidence That Does Not Support the Hot Thought	6. Alternative/ Balanced Thoughts	7. Rate Moods Now
		a. Write an alternative or balanced thought. b. Rate how much you believe in each alternative or balanced thought (0–100%).	Rerate moods listed in column 2 as well as any new moods (0–100%).
I'm so empty inside. I just have to die. The pain is unbearable. Killing myself is the only way to get rid of the pain. I've tried many types of psychotherapy, many therapists, and many medications, which haven't helped.			

Figure 6.4 reflects the information Marissa gathered with her therapist's help.

THOUGHT

1. Situation	2. Moods	3. Automatic Thoughts (Images)
Who? What? When? Where?	a. What did you feel? b. Rate each mood (0–100%).	a. What was going though your mind just before you started to feel this way? Any other thoughts? Images? b. Circle the hot thought.
At home alone, Saturday, 9:30 P.M.	Depressed 100% Disappointed 95% Empty 100% Confused 90% Unreal 95%	I want to go numb so I don't have to feel anymore. I'm not making any progress. I'm so confused that I can't think clearly. I don't know what's real and what isn't. (The pain is so great that I have to kill myself.) Nothing helps. Life is not worth living. I'm such a failure. I'm so empty inside.

FIGURE 6.4. Marissa's Thought Record with complete evidence.

RECORD

4. Evidence That Supports the Hot Thought	5. Evidence That Does Not Support the Hot Thought	6. Alternative/ Balanced Thoughts a. Write an alternative or balanced thought. b. Rate how much you believe in each alternative or balanced thought (0–100%).	7. Rate Moods Now Rerate moods listed in column 2 as well as any new moods (0–100%).
I just have to die. The pain is unbearable. Killing myself is the only way to get rid of the pain. I've tried many types of psychotherapy, many therapists, and many medications, which haven't helped.	In the past, talking about my feelings sometimes helped me feel better. I have felt suicidal and in severe emotional pain in the past and have gotten through it every time. I'm learning to think differently, which might help, although I'm doubtful. Kate sees me as having positive qualities and a lot to contribute to the world. Some days I feel better and in less emotional pain. I laugh occasionally.		

It is important to *write down* the evidence you uncover while answering the questions in the Hint Box on page 70. Marissa remained quite hopeless while discussing this evidence with her therapist. But when she wrote it down on her Thought Record, she discovered that seeing it all at once did make her feel somewhat more hopeful and less depressed. Similarly, you will benefit more from writing down the evidence in your own life rather than simply thinking about it.

REMINDER BOX

- To complete column 5 of a Thought Record, ask yourself the questions in the Hint Box on page 70.

- *Write down* all the evidence that shows that your hot thought is not completely true rather than simply thinking about it.

THOUGHT

1. Situation	2. Moods	3. Automatic Thoughts (Images)
Who? What? When? Where?	**a.** What did you feel? **b.** Rate each mood (0–100%).	**a.** What was going though your mind just before you started to feel this way? Any other thoughts? Images? **b.** Circle the hot thought.
Sunday evening, in the airplane, on the runway, waiting for the plane to take off.	Fear 98%	I'm feeling sick. My heart is starting to beat harder and faster. I'm starting to sweat. I'm having a heart attack. I'll never be able to get off this plane and to a hospital in time. I'm going to die.

FIGURE 6.5.   Linda's partially completed Thought Record.

LINDA: *Untruth or consequences.*

As her treatment progressed, Linda became more skilled at asking herself the questions that allowed her to complete column 5 of the Thought Record. This skill became an important component in Linda's overall ability to prevent her anxiety symptoms from escalating into a panic attack. Figure 6.5 demonstrates how Linda began to regain control by listing in column 4 in the Thought Record the evidence in support of her hottest automatic thought as she was waiting for a flight to take off.

Then Linda began to gather evidence that did not support her hot thought. As she was sitting on the airplane, Linda thought about what her best friend might tell her if she were sitting next to her. She knew that her friend would tell her that her rapid heartbeat was probably caused by her

RECORD

4. Evidence That Supports the Hot Thought	5. Evidence That Does Not Support the Hot Thought	6. Alternative/ Balanced Thoughts a. Write an alternative or balanced thought. b. Rate how much you believe in each alternative or balanced thought (0–100%).	7. Rate Moods Now Rerate moods listed in column 2 as well as any new moods (0–100%).
My heart is racing. I'm sweating. These are two characteristics of a heart attack.			

nervousness and anxiety and did not necessarily mean that she was having a heart attack. Further, Linda remembered that her physician had told her that her heart was a muscle and making it beat faster was not dangerous. He reassured her that a rapid heartbeat is not dangerous nor is it a definite sign of a heart attack.

Linda also asked herself whether she had had any experiences that demonstrated that her hot thought was not true. She realized that, in fact, she had had a rapid heartbeat many times before on airplanes, in airports, and when thinking about flying. Even though she had believed that she was having a heart attack in those situations, she understood now that she was having a panic attack, not a heart attack.

THOUGHT

1. Situation	2. Moods	3. Automatic Thoughts (Images)
Who? What? When? Where?	**a.** What did you feel? **b.** Rate each mood (0–100%).	**a.** What was going though your mind just before you started to feel this way? Any other thoughts? Images? **b.** Circle the hot thought.
Sunday evening, in the airplane, on the runway, waiting for the plane to take off.	Fear 98%	I'm feeling sick. My heart is starting to beat harder and faster. I'm starting to sweat. ⬭I'm having a heart attack.⬭ I'll never be able to get off this plane and to a hospital in time. I'm going to die.

FIGURE 6.6. Linda's Thought Record with complete evidence.

Finally, Linda asked herself what she had done or thought about in the past that had helped her feel better. She remembered that she had been helped in the past by concentrating on reading a magazine, breathing deeply, doing Thought Records, and thinking in ways that were noncatastrophic. As she asked herself the questions from the Hint Box on page 70, Linda wrote her answers down in column 5 at Figure 6.6.

The questions and answers enabled Linda to attend to important information that contradicted her initial conclusion that she was having a heart attack. If Linda considered this information, her anxiety decreased.

RECORD

4. Evidence That Supports the Hot Thought	5. Evidence That Does Not Support the Hot Thought	6. Alternative/ Balanced Thoughts a. Write an alternative or balanced thought. b. Rate how much you believe in each alternative or balanced thought (0–100%).	7. Rate Moods Now Rerate moods listed in column 2 as well as any new moods (0–100%).
My heart is racing. I'm sweating. These are two characteristics of a heart attack.	A rapid heartbeat can be characteristic of anxiety. My doctor told me that the heart is a muscle, using a muscle is not dangerous, and therefore a rapid heartbeat is not dangerous. A rapid heartbeat doesn't mean that I am having a heart attack. I have had this happen to me before in airports, on airplanes, and when thinking about flying. In the past my heartbeat has returned to normal when I read a magazine, practiced deep breathing, did Thought Records, or thought in noncatastrophic ways.		

EXERCISE: Identifying Evidence That Supports and Contradicts Hot Thoughts

Just as Linda asked the questions from the Box on page 70 to help her gather evidence that did not support her hot thought, so can you use the same questions to test the hot thoughts you identified on your Thought Records at the end of Chapter 5. Look back at these Thought Records now. Choose two or three to continue completing here. Alternatively, if you do not want to continue the Thought Records you began in Chapter 5, identify two or three situations in which you recently had strong feelings and complete Worksheets 6.1 for them.

On each Thought Record circle the hot thought that you will test on Worksheet 6.1. In columns 4 and 5 of the Thought Record, list information that supports and contradicts the circled hot thought.

WORKSHEET 6.1: Where's the Evidence?

THOUGHT

1. Situation	2. Moods	3. Automatic Thoughts (Images)
		Answer some or all of the following questions: What was going through my mind just before I started to feel this way? What does this say about me? What does this mean about me? my life? my future? What am I afraid might happen? What is the worst thing that could happen if this is true? What does this mean about how the other person(s) feel(s)/think(s) about me? What does this mean about the other person(s) or people in general? What images or memories do I have in this situation?
Who were you with? What were you doing? When was it? Where were you?	Describe each mood in one word. Rate intensity of mood (0–100%).	

Try to list in column 4 only factual evidence that supports the hot thought, not interpretations of facts or mind reading. For example, "Peter stared at me" is an example of factual evidence. The statement, "Peter stared at me and thought I was crazy" would not be factual unless Peter had actually said aloud, "I think you are crazy." If Peter had been staring silently, your assumption that you knew what he was thinking is mind reading.

Once you have completed column 4, ask yourself the questions in the Box on page 70 to look for evidence that does not support your hot thought. Write down each piece of evidence you uncover in column 5. Completing the two Evidence columns of the Thought Record allows you to evaluate your hot thought in the light of several perspectives.

RECORD

4. Evidence That Supports the Hot Thought	5. Evidence That Does Not Support the Hot Thought	6. Alternative/ Balanced Thoughts	7. Rate Moods Now
Circle hot thought in previous column for which you are looking for evidence. Write factual evidence to support this conclusion. (Try to avoid mind-reading and interpretation of facts.)	Ask yourself the questions in the Hint Box (p. 70) to help discover evidence which does not support your hot thought.		

Chapter 7 will teach you what you need to know to complete the last two columns of the Thought Record. Before proceeding to the next chapter, complete the first five columns on five or six Thought Records. You can start with partially completed Thought Records from Chapter 5 (Worksheet 5.3)

WORKSHEET 6.1: Where's the Evidence?

THOUGHT

1. Situation	2. Moods	3. Automatic Thoughts (Images)
		Answer some or all of the following questions: What was going through my mind just before I started to feel this way? What does this say about me? What does this mean about me? my life? my future? What am I afraid might happen? What is the worst thing that could happen if this is true? What does this mean about how the other person(s) feel(s)/think(s) about me? What does this mean about the other person(s) or people in general?
Who were you with? What were you doing? When was it? Where were you?	Describe each mood in one word. Rate intensity of mood (0–100%).	What image or memories do I have in this situation?

and/or begin Thought Records for more recent situations (Worksheet 6.1). The more you practice looking for evidence for and against hot thoughts, the more quickly you will develop the type of flexible thinking that is linked to feeling better.

RECORD

4. Evidence That Supports the Hot Thought	5. Evidence That Does Not Support the Hot Thought	6. Alternative/ Balanced Thoughts a. Write an alternative or balanced thought. b. Rate how much you believe in each alternative or balanced thought (0–100%).	7. Rate Moods Now Rerate moods listed in column 2 as well as any new moods (0–100%).
Circle hot thought in previous column for which you are looking for evidence. Write factual evidence to support this conclusion. (Try to avoid mind-reading and interpretation of facts.)	Ask yourself the questions in the Hint Box (p. 70) to help discover evidence your hot thought is not completely true.		

WORKSHEET 6.1:   Where's the Evidence?

THOUGHT

1. Situation	2. Moods	3. Automatic Thoughts (Images)
		Answer some or all of the following questions: What was going through my mind just before I started to feel this way? What does this say about me? What does this mean about me? my life? my future? What am I afraid might happen? What is the worst thing that could happen if this is true? What does this mean about how the other person(s) feel(s)/think(s) about me? What does this mean about the other person(s) or people in general? What images or memories do I have in this situation?
Who were you with? What were you doing? When was it? Where were you?	Describe each mood in one word. Rate intensity of mood (0–100%).	

RECORD

4. Evidence That Supports the Hot Thought	5. Evidence That Does Not Support the Hot Thought	6. Alternative/ Balanced Thoughts a. Write an alternative or balanced thought. b. Rate how much you believe in each alternative or balanced thought (0–100%).	7. Rate Moods Now Rerate moods listed in column 2 as well as any new moods (0–100%).
Circle hot thought in previous column for which you are looking for evidence. Write factual evidence to support this conclusion. (Try to avoid mind-reading and interpretation of facts.)	Ask yourself the questions in the Hint Box (p. 70) to help discover evidence your hot thought is not completely true.		

WORKSHEET 6.1: Where's the Evidence?

THOUGHT

1. Situation	2. Moods	3. Automatic Thoughts (Images)
		Answer some or all of the following questions: What was going through my mind just before I started to feel this way? What does this say about me? What does this mean about me? my life? my future? What am I afraid might happen? What is the worst thing that could happen if this is true? What does this mean about how the other person(s) feel(s)/think(s) about me? What does this mean about the other person(s) or people in general? What images or memories do I have in this situation?
Who were you with? What were you doing? When was it? Where were you?	Describe each mood in one word. Rate intensity of mood (0–100%).	

RECORD

4. Evidence That Supports the Hot Thought	5. Evidence That Does Not Support the Hot Thought	6. Alternative/ Balanced Thoughts	7. Rate Moods Now
		a. Write an alternative or balanced thought. **b.** Rate how much you believe in each alternative or balanced thought (0– 100%).	Rerate moods listed in column 2 as well as any new moods (0–100%).
Circle hot thought in previous column for which you are looking for evidence. Write factual evidence to support this conclusion. (Try to avoid mind-reading and interpretation of facts.)	Ask yourself the questions in the Hint Box (p. 70) to help discover evidence your hot thought is not completely true.		

CHAPTER 6 SUMMARY

- When we have negative automatic thoughts, we usually dwell on data that confirm our conclusions.

- It is helpful to consider your hot thoughts as hypotheses or guesses.

- Gathering evidence that supports and does not support your hot thoughts can help clarify your thinking and reduce the intensity of distressing moods.

- Evidence consists of data, information, and facts, not interpretations.

- Column 5 of the Thought Record asks you to actively search for information that contradicts your hot thoughts.

- You can ask yourself the specific questions in the Hint Box on page 70 to help you complete column 5 of a Thought Record.

- It is important to write down all evidence that may demonstrate that your hot thought is not 100% true.

- Considering information that contradicts your hot thought can help you feel better.

CHAPTER 7

Alternative or Balanced Thinking

Sally was at home with the flu and asked her 7-year-old daughter, Barbara, to play quietly while she rested. An hour later, Sally walked into the kitchen to get a drink of water and was distressed to see crayons spread all over the floor, shredded colored paper and an open bottle of glue on the table, open scissors in the wastebasket, and a half-drunk glass of milk on the counter next to the refrigerator.

Furious about the mess, Sally went hunting for Barbara and found her sleeping soundly in front of the television in the living room. On the cushion near Barbara's head was a large, brightly colored card, covered in hearts, that read, "I love you, Mom! Please get well soon!" Sally shook her head slowly and smiled. She tucked a blanket around Barbara's shoulders and returned to the kitchen to get her water.

Sometimes a little bit of additional information shifts our interpretation of a situation 180 degrees. When Sally first walked into the kitchen, she was not expecting a mess and immediately felt angry that Barbara had made one, especially when Sally was sick. Sally's hot thought accompanying her anger was "Barbara is so inconsiderate to make such a mess when she knows I'm sick."

When Sally discovered the beautiful get-well card, her emotional response shifted immediately. Sally thought, "Barbara was concerned for me and wanted to help me feel better—how thoughtful!" Feelings of appreciation and tenderness toward Barbara followed this alternative thought. Learning the meaning behind the mess led to a shift in Sally's attitude and mood.

VIC: *Gathering new evidence.*

Chapter 6 began with a description of Vic's reaction to the change in his wife Judy's facial expression when he told her he had plans to attend a Saturday AA meeting. Vic's interpretation of Judy's facial expression was "She's upset that I'm spending time away from her and the kids." His anger was fueled by further thoughts: "It's not fair that she doesn't see my recovery program as important," "If she cared about me as much as the kids, she'd be happy I was going to AA," and "She doesn't care about me."

Vic's interpretation of Judy's expression led to a behavioral as well as an emotional response. He yelled at Judy, slammed his fist on the table, stormed out of the house, and drove to a nearby bar. Fortunately, before going into the bar, Vic completed a Thought Record that looked for evidence both supporting and not supporting his hot thought, "She doesn't care about me" (Figure 6.1).

As Vic considered all the information on his Thought Record, he realized that Judy did seem to care for him in many important ways. In fact, he began to wonder why she would be so upset about his plan to attend an AA meeting. Vic's therapist had pointed out that Vic's distress at work often followed instances where Vic made assumptions about what his supervisor was thinking (mind reading)—assumptions that were often wrong. Vic began to wonder whether he was wrong in his assumption about what Judy was thinking.

Instead of getting a drink in the bar, Vic decided to call his AA sponsor. After talking for a few minutes, the sponsor advised Vic to go to a local AA meeting before heading home. After the meeting, when Vic went home, he found Judy anxiously waiting for him.

As Vic and Judy began to talk about their argument, Vic decided to test his assumptions by asking Judy about her reaction when he told her he had made plans to go to the AA meeting on Saturday. Judy's response surprised Vic. She said that when he mentioned Saturday, she had remembered that that day was her sister's birthday, and she had forgotten to mail a card. Judy had been concerned that her sister would be upset or hurt if a card didn't arrive on time. Judy had not been aware of a change in facial expression, but if it had changed, she was certain that these were the thoughts that had caused it—she hadn't been thinking about Vic at all!

Vic sheepishly told Judy that he had thought her look meant that she was upset with him for planning to attend a meeting on Saturday, and that he had been angry because he thought this meant that she didn't care about him or his sobriety. Judy voiced her support for Vic's recovery program and told him that she had worried while he was gone that he would drink and be killed driving. She said she loved him very much although his quick anger was becoming increasingly difficult for her to tolerate. Vic sincerely apologized and vowed to try to spot and stop his mind reading.

♦   ♦   ♦

Both Sally's change in mood when she saw the get-well card and Vic's realization that his wife's facial expression did not pertain to him illustrate how additional information can shift one's perspective of a distressing situation. Vic and Sally each discovered an alternative explanation for events that was less distressing than their original interpretation. Vic and Sally each felt better after gathering evidence and arriving at an interpretation based on evidence.

In Chapter 6 you learned to ask yourself questions to actively look for evidence that supports and contradicts your hottest thoughts (Hint Box, p. 70). Sometimes the evidence you find will show that your hot thoughts are not very accurate. Sally discovered that her 7-year-old daughter was not being inconsiderate, and Vic found out that his wife's facial expression was not a negative reaction to him. When the evidence in columns 4 and 5 of the Thought Record does not support your original automatic thought, write an alternative explanation for the situation in column 6, as illustrated in Figure 7.1 on the following two pages.

Notice that Vic rated his belief in his alternative thoughts very high. He completely believed that Judy's change in facial expression was due to remembering her sister's birthday and so he rated his belief in this alternative thought as 100%. He was also completely confident after their discussion that Judy supported his AA attendance and wanted him to stay sober. Vic rated his belief in the last alternative thought, that Judy cared about him, as 80%. He strongly believed she cared but still reserved some doubt. The alternative view(s) of a situation you write should put all the evidence you gathered in perspective.

THOUGHT

1. Situation	2. Moods	3. Automatic Thoughts (Images)
Who? What? When? Where?	**a.** What did you feel? **b.** Rate each mood (0–100%).	**a.** What was going though your mind just before you started to feel this way? Any other thoughts? Images? **b.** Circle the hot thought.
Thursday, 8:30 P.M. Judy gives me an odd look when I tell her I'm going to AA on Saturday	*Anger 90%*	*She's upset that I'm going to AA on Saturday.* *She doesn't see my recovery program as important.* *She doesn't care about me.* *She doesn't understand how hard it is not to drink.* *I can't stand being so angry. A drink will make me feel better.*

FIGURE 7.1. Vic's Thought Record.

RECORD

4. Evidence That Supports the Hot Thought	5. Evidence That Does Not Support the Hot Thought	6. Alternative/ Balanced Thoughts	7. Rate Moods Now
		a. Write an alternative or balanced thought. b. Rate how much you believe in each alternative or balanced thought (0–100%).	Rerate moods listed in column 2 as well as any new moods (0–100%).
She's not supportive of AA. She nags me to do things. She doesn't seem to appreciate how hard I work. She's always giving me negative looks like tonight. She yelled at me as I was leaving the house.	She stuck with me during all those years of drinking. She attended Al-Anon meetings for a year. She seemed happy to see me when I came home from work tonight. She tells me she loves me and does nice things for me when we're not fighting. Judy explained that her facial expression was due to remembering her sister's birthday. Judy says she is glad I am in AA and she wants me to go to meetings.	The look on Judy's face was because she remembered her sister's birthday. 100% She is supportive of my AA attendance and wants me to stay sober. 100% She does care about me. 80%	

Rating your belief in the alternative view(s) helps you see how much the additional evidence you gathered leads to a credible alternative view.

Vic's perspective changed almost completely. He shifted from a belief that Judy didn't care to one that she did. Sometimes the evidence does not lead to a total shift in perspective. Often the new view of a situation will be more of a balanced perspective (based on the evidence that supports and contradicts your original conclusion) than a totally different alternative view.

To construct a balanced thought, it helps to write one sentence that summarizes column 4 of the Thought Record and a second sentence that summarizes column 5, then, if appropriate, connect the two sentences with the word "and." For example, after examining the evidence, a more balanced thought for someone who originally concludes "I'm a bad parent," might be "I've made some mistakes as a parent and done some good things, too." This statement is probably a more balanced view of all the person's parenting experiences than the original conclusion, "I'm a bad parent," which focuses only on negative parenting experiences.

To summarize, column 6 of the Thought Record should include either an alternative view of the original situation or a balanced thought that summarizes as fairly as possible the evidence in columns 4 and 5. Either the alternative view or the balanced thought in column 6 should be consistent with the evidence summarized in columns 4 and 5. Questions you can ask yourself to help arrive at a balanced or alternative thought appear in the Hint Box on the facing page.

REMINDER BOX

ALTERNATIVE OR BALANCED THINKING

Column 6 of the Thought Record should summarize the important evidence collected and recorded in columns 4 and 5.

1. If the evidence does *not* support your automatic thought(s), write an alternative view of the situation that is consistent with the evidence.

2. If the evidence only partially supports your automatic thought(s), write a balanced thought that summarizes the evidence supporting and contradicting your original thought.

3. Rate your belief in the new alternative or balanced thought on a 0–100% scale.

Alternative or balanced thinking often emerges from an expanded view of yourself or of the situation you are in. Alternative or balanced thinking is often more positive than the initial automatic thought, but it is not merely the substitution of a positive thought for a negative thought. It is important to differentiate and contrast alternative or balanced thinking with merely thinking in a more positive way. Positive thinking tends to ignore negative information and can be as damaging as negative thinking. Alternative or balanced thinking takes into account both negative and positive information. It is an attempt to understand the meaning of *all* the available information. With additional information or an expanded point of view, your interpretation of an event may change.

HELPFUL HINTS

☞

QUESTIONS TO HELP ARRIVE AT ALTERNATIVE OR BALANCED THINKING

- Based on the evidence I have listed in columns 4 and 5 of the Thought Record, is there an alternative way of thinking about or understanding this situation?

- Write one sentence that summarizes all the evidence that supports my hot thought (column 4) and all the evidence that does not support my hot thought (column 5). Does combining the two summary statements with the word "and" create a balanced thought that takes into account all the information I have gathered?

- If someone I cared about was in this situation, had these thoughts, and had this information available, what would be my advice to them? How would I suggest that they understand the situation?

- If my hot thought is true, what is the worst outcome? If my hot thought is true, what is the best outcome? If my hot thought is true, what is the most realistic outcome?

- Can someone I trust think of any other way of understanding this situation?

From *Mind Over Mood* by Dennis Greenberger and Christine A. Padesky. © 1995 The Guilford Press.

Column 7 of the Thought Record asks you to rerate the moods you identified in column 2. If you have constructed a balanced/alternative thought that is believable, you will probably notice that the intensity of your uncomfortable feelings has diminished.

The following examples demonstrate how Marissa, Ben, and Linda developed alternative or balanced thoughts and completed columns 6 and 7 of their Thought Records. The examples complete the Thought Records begun in Chapter 6 (Figures 6.2, 6.4, and 6.6).

BEN: *Balanced thinking.*

Ben, in Chapter 6, brought to therapy a Thought Record regarding his experiences on Thanksgiving Day (Figure 6.2). Ben identified his hot automatic thought as "The kids and grandkids don't need me anymore. They didn't

pay any attention to me all day." Ben then gathered evidence that supported and did not support his hot thought. After writing the evidence in
columns 4 and 5 of the Thought Record, Ben reviewed the questions in the
Hint Box on page 95 to help construct a balanced thought for column 6.

Ben pondered the questions in the Hint Box while he studied the evidence in columns 4 and 5. He concluded that the evidence did not consis-

THOUGHT

1. Situation	2. Moods	3. Automatic Thoughts (Images)
Who? What? When? Where?	**a.** What did you feel? **b.** Rate each mood (0–100%).	**a.** What was going though your mind just be-fore you started to feel this way? Any other thoughts? Images? **b.** Circle the hot thought.
November 25, 9:00 P.M. Driving home from my daughter's home where I spent Thanksgiving with my daughter, son-in-law, two of my grandchildren, and my wife.	*Sad 80%*	*They all would have had a better time if I hadn't been there today.* *The kids and grandkids don't need me anymore.* *They didn't pay any attention to me all day.*

FIGURE 7.2. Ben's Thought Record.

tently support his hottest thought. Ben decided that a more accurate and balanced way of understanding the experience was "Even though my children and grandchildren don't need me in the same ways they used to, they still enjoy my company and they still ask for my advice. They paid attention to me throughout the day, although the attention was not as consistent or the same as it has been in the past." After Ben wrote this balanced thought, he noticed that the intensity rating of his sadness lessened from 80% to 30%. His completed Thought Record is shown in Figure 7.2.

RECORD

4. Evidence That Supports the Hot Thought	5. Evidence That Does Not Support the Hot Thought	6. Alternative/ Balanced Thoughts a. Write an alternative or balanced thought. b. Rate how much you believe in each alternative or balanced thought (0–100%).	7. Rate Moods Now Rerate moods listed in column 2 as well as any new moods (0–100%).
I used to enjoy tying my granddaughter's shoes, but now she wants to do this on her own. My daughter and son-in-law have their lives together and they don't need anything from me. Amy, the 15-year-old, left at 7:00 P.M. to be with her friends. Bill, my son-in-law, built new shelves and cabinets in the family room. Three years ago he would have asked me and needed me to help him with a project that big.	Bill asked for my advice on plans for a room addition to their home. My daughter asked me to take a look at some vegetables in their garden that were dying. I was able to tell her that they weren't getting enough water. I made my 5-year-old granddaughter laugh often throughout the day. Sally seemed to enjoy my stories about her mom as a teenager. My five-year-old granddaughter fell asleep in my lap.	Even though my children and grandchildren don't need me in the same ways they used to, they still enjoy my company and they still ask for my advice. 85% They paid attention to me throughout the day although the attention was not as consistent or the same as it has been in the past. 90%	Sad 30%

If Ben had simply substituted a positive thought, he might have concluded, "They need me more than they ever have." If he had attempted to merely rationalize away his sadness, he might have decided, "They don't need me anymore, but what do I care?" Positive thinking and rationalization can lead to problems. For Ben, positive thinking would have ignored real changes that were taking place in his family; rationalization could have led Ben to feel even more isolated and alone. In contrast, Ben's balanced thought emerged from the evidence and allowed Ben to understand his experience in a way that lessened his sadness and increased his connection to his family.

Further, notice that Ben's balanced thought is plausible and believable. The more an alternative or balanced thought is believable to you, the more it will relieve the intensity of your negative feelings. If you simply provide a rationalization or a positive thought that you do not believe, it is not likely to have a lasting impact.

Marissa: *Alternative thinking.*

In Chapter 6, Marissa described an experience in which she felt depressed, disappointed, empty, confused, and unreal (Figure 6.4). She identified numerous automatic thoughts and determined that the hot thought was "The pain is so great that I have to kill myself." Marissa completed columns 4 and 5 of the Thought Record with the help of her therapist. To complete column 6, Marissa reviewed the questions in the Hint Box (p. 95) with her therapist. The question that was most relevant for Marissa was "If Kate was in this situation, had these thoughts, and had this information available, how would I suggest that she understand the situation?" Marissa concluded that she would suggest to Kate, "Even though the emotional pain is severe, in the past talking has helped you to feel better. It's important to recognize that this unbearable feeling won't last and that you will feel better later. Suicide is not the only solution—you are learning new skills that may help you break old patterns." Marissa's completed Thought Record is shown in Figure 7.3 on pages 100 and 101.

It was easier for Marissa to think of alternatives to suicide when she imagined the advice she would give to Kate. By doing this she was able to distance herself from her own life and find a different perspective. She was able to see that there was an alternative way of thinking in the situation. Even though the alternative thoughts were only slightly believable to Marissa, they still made a small, positive difference in how she felt. Even this small change had an important effect on Marissa's desire to kill herself. The therapist reminded her that she had had the automatic thoughts and feelings for a long time, so even small changes could be interpreted as encouraging and hopeful.

The amount of change you notice in your moods when you rerate them in column 7 will probably vary with how much you believe your alternative or balanced thoughts. Since Marissa believed her alternative thoughts only slightly (ratings of 10–20%), her feelings did not change dramatically. Over time, if her alternative views match her experiences Marissa's moods will shift more as the hope for improvement becomes more believable.

Recall that Ben rated his sadness 80% when he was driving home from his daughter's home thinking, "The kids and grandkids don't need me anymore. They didn't pay any attention to me all day." After constructing the balanced thought "Even though my children and grandchildren don't need me in the same ways they used to, they still enjoy my company and ask for my advice," Ben's sadness rating dropped to 30%.

Ben's sadness did not disappear completely after he completed a Thought Record, even though his balanced thought was highly believable (85%) to him. Some sadness remained because some of the evidence pointed to changes that Ben was experiencing as losses. The goal of a Thought Record is not to eliminate emotions. Instead, the Thought Record is designed to help you gain a broader perspective on a situation so that your emotional reactions are balanced responses to the total circumstances of your life.

If your Thought Record was completed properly and your mood did not change, your hot thought may be a core belief (see Chapter 9 for additional ideas for shifting core beliefs). Perhaps your hot thought is accurate. If so, an action plan needs to be developed and implemented before your moods will decrease (Chapter 8 helps you develop action plans).

THOUGHT

1. Situation	2. Moods	3. Automatic Thoughts (Images)
Who? What? When? Where?	a. What did you feel? b. Rate each mood (0–100%).	a. What was going though your mind just before you started to feel this way? Any other thoughts? Images? b. Circle the hot thought.
At home, alone, Saturday, 9:30 P.M.	*Depressed* *100%* *Disappointed* *95%* *Empty* *100%* *Confused* *90%* *Unreal* *95%*	*I want to go numb so I don't have to feel anymore.* *I'm not making any progress.* *I'm so confused that I can't think clearly.* *I don't know what's real and what isn't.* *The pain is so great that I have to kill myself.* *Nothing helps.* *Life is not worth living.* *I'm such a failure.* *I'm so empty inside.* *I just have to die.*

Figure 7.3. Marissa's Thought Record.

RECORD

4. Evidence That Supports the Hot Thought	5. Evidence That Does Not Support the Hot Thought	6. Alternative/ Balanced Thoughts a. Write an alternative or balanced thought. b. Rate how much you believe in each alternative or balanced thought (0–100%).	7. Rate Moods Now Rerate moods listed in column 2 as well as any new moods (0–100%).
The pain is unbearable. Killing myself is the only way to get rid of the pain. I've tried many types of psychotherapy, many therapists and many medications which haven't helped.	In the past, talking about my feelings sometimes helped me feel better. I have felt suicidal and in severe emotional pain in the past and have gotten through it every time. I'm learning to think differently, which might help, although I'm doubtful. Kate sees me as having positive qualities and a lot to contribute to the world. Some days I feel better and in less pain. I laugh occasionally.	Even though the emotional pain is severe talking might help me feel better as it did in the past. 15% It is important to recognize that this unbearable feeling won't last and I will feel better again. 10% Suicide is not the only solution. 20% I am learning new skills that may help break old patterns. 15%	Depressed 85% Disappointed 90% Empty 95% Confused 85% Unreal 95%

What should you think or do if there is no shift in emotional response after you complete a Thought Record? First review your Thought Record to make sure you completed it properly. The following Troubleshooting Guide lists questions to ask yourself if there has been no change in your moods after you have completed a Thought Record.

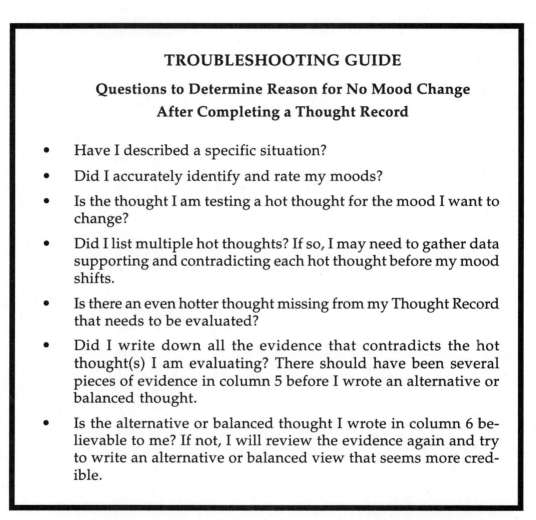

TROUBLESHOOTING GUIDE

**Questions to Determine Reason for No Mood Change
After Completing a Thought Record**

- Have I described a specific situation?

- Did I accurately identify and rate my moods?

- Is the thought I am testing a hot thought for the mood I want to change?

- Did I list multiple hot thoughts? If so, I may need to gather data supporting and contradicting each hot thought before my mood shifts.

- Is there an even hotter thought missing from my Thought Record that needs to be evaluated?

- Did I write down all the evidence that contradicts the hot thought(s) I am evaluating? There should have been several pieces of evidence in column 5 before I wrote an alternative or balanced thought.

- Is the alternative or balanced thought I wrote in column 6 believable to me? If not, I will review the evidence again and try to write an alternative or balanced view that seems more credible.

It is sometimes easier to recognize alternative ways of seeing situations for other people than for ourselves. In Chapter 6, Linda wrote out a Thought Record for her experience of fear while sitting in an airplane on a runway awaiting takeoff (Figure 6.6). Her partially completed Thought Record is duplicated on Worksheet 7.1 on pages 104 and 105.

EXERCISE: Helping Linda Arrive at an Alternative or Balanced Thought

In columns 4 and 5 Linda wrote down evidence that supported and contradicted the hot thought "I'm having a heart attack." Based on this evidence, write in column 6 of Worksheet 7.1 a believable alternative or balanced thought that would reduce Linda's fear. If you have difficulty completing this exercise, refer to the Hint Box on page 95 for suggestions. Complete column 6 on Worksheet 7.1 before reading further.

Linda herself, in completing column 6, studied the evidence she had gathered in columns 4 and 5 and considered numerous alternatives to her hot thought. The evidence suggested that she was not having a heart attack but that her rapid heartbeat and sweating were caused by her anxiety and were in no way dangerous or harmful to her. Instead of thinking, "I'm having a heart attack," Linda concluded, "My heart is racing and I am sweating because I'm anxious/nervous about being on an airplane. My doctor assured me that a rapid heartbeat is not necessarily dangerous, and in all likelihood my heartbeat will return to normal in just a few minutes." Linda's completed Thought Record which she finished while she was still on the runway, is shown in Figure 7.4 on pages 106 and 107.

As Linda changed the meaning she attached to her rapid heartbeat and sweating, her fear dropped considerably. Her fear had been connected to the thought "I'm having a heart attack." By examining the evidence for and against that thought and concluding that she was not having a heart attack, Linda's fear was substantially reduced.

WORKSHEET 7.1: Completing Linda's Thought Record

THOUGHT

1. Situation	2. Moods	3. Automatic Thoughts (Images)
Who? What? When? Where?	a. What did you feel? b. Rate each mood (0–100%).	a. What was going though your mind just before you started to feel this way? Any other thoughts? Images? b. Circle the hot thought.
Sunday evening, in the airplane, on the runway, waiting for the plane to take off.	Fear 98%	I'm feeling sick. My heart is starting to beat harder and faster. I'm starting to sweat. ⟨I'm having a heart attack.⟩ I'll never be able to get off this plane and to a hospital in time. I'm going to die.

RECORD

4. Evidence That Supports the Hot Thought	5. Evidence That Does Not Support the Hot Thought	6. Alternative/ Balanced Thoughts a. Write an alternative or balanced thought. b. Rate how much you believe in each alternative or balanced thought (0–100%).	7. Rate Moods Now Rerate moods listed in column 2 as well as any new moods (0–100%).
My heart is racing. I'm sweating. These are two characteristics of a heart attack.	A rapid heartbeat can be characteristic of anxiety. My doctor told me that the heart is a muscle, using a muscle is not dangerous, and therefore a rapid heartbeat is not dangerous. A rapid heartbeat doesn't mean that I am having a heart attack. I have had this happen to me before in airports, on airplanes and when thinking about flying. In the past, my heartbeat has returned to normal when I read a magazine, practiced deep breathing, did Thought Records, or thought in non-catastrophic ways.		

THOUGHT

1. Situation	2. Moods	3. Automatic Thoughts (Images)
Who? What? When? Where?	**a.** What did you feel? **b.** Rate each mood (0–100%).	**a.** What was going though your mind just before you started to feel this way? Any other thoughts? Images? **b.** Circle the hot thought.
Sunday evening, in the airplane, on the runway, waiting for the plane to take off.	*Fear 98%*	*I'm feeling sick.* *My heart is starting to beat harder and faster.* *I'm starting to sweat.* *(I'm having a heart attack.)* *I'll never be able to get off this plane and to a hospital in time.* *I'm going to die.*

Figure 7.4. Linda's completed Thought Record.

RECORD

4. Evidence That Supports the Hot Thought	5. Evidence That Does Not Support the Hot Thought	6. Alternative/ Balanced Thoughts a. Write an alternative or balanced thought. b. Rate how much you believe in each alternative or balanced thought (0–100%).	7. Rate Moods Now Rerate moods listed in column 2 as well as any new moods (0–100%).
My heart is racing. I'm sweating. These are two characteristics of a heart attack.	A rapid heartbeat can be characteristic of anxiety. My doctor told me that the heart is a muscle, using a muscle is not dangerous, and therefore a rapid heartbeat is not dangerous. A rapid heartbeat doesn't mean that I am having a heart attack. I have had this happen to me before in airports, on airplanes and when thinking about flying. In the past, my heartbeat has returned to normal when I read a magazine, practiced deep breathing, did Thought Records, or thought in non-catastrophic ways.	My heart is racing and I am sweating because I'm anxious and nervous about being on an airplane. 95% My doctor assured me that a rapid heartbeat is not necessarily dangerous and in all likelihood my heart will return to normal in just a few minutes. 85%	Fear 25%

**Exercises: Constructing Your Own
Alternative or Balanced Thoughts**

Just as you looked at the evidence on Linda's Thought Record and constructed an alternative or balanced belief, on Worksheet 7.2 do the same for the Thought Records you completed in Chapter 6 (Worksheet 6.1).

First, use the questions in the Hint Box (p. 95) to help construct an alternative or balanced thought for the hot thought circled on each Thought Record. Write the alternative or balanced thought in column 6 of the Thought Records. Now rate the believability of your alternative or balanced thoughts on a scale of 0–100%. Write the rating next to the thought in column 6.

Rerate your mood(s) after you have written the alternative or balanced thought. Write the mood(s) and rating(s) in column 7. Is there a relationship between the believability of your alternative or balanced thought and the change in your emotional response? If your mood has not changed for the better, use the Troubleshooting Guide on page 102 to try to understand why your mood is the same or worse, and try to improve your Thought Record so that it more effectively helps to reduce your emotional distress.

Now you have learned what you need to know to complete all seven columns of a Thought Record. In doing Thought Records, you identify and alter the thinking and beliefs that contribute to your emotional distress. Constructing alternative or balanced thoughts helps free you from automatic thinking patterns that contribute to the difficulties you are having. If you are able to see yourself and situations from a different perspective, it is possible that you will begin to feel better about yourself and your life.

Complete two or three Thought Records per week to help improve your skills in developing alternative and balanced thinking. (There are blank Thought Records in the Appendix to this book.) In the future, whenever you get stuck evaluating a thought, you can write down the evidence in a Thought Record.

There are two advantages to completing Thought Records regularly. First, a Thought Record can help you broaden your perspective on troubling situations so that you react in ways that are consistent with the big picture rather than a narrow and possibly distorted view. Second, Thought Records actually help you learn to think automatically in more flexible ways. After completing 20 to 50 Thought Records, many people report that they begin to think alternative or balanced thoughts in distressing situations without writing out a Thought Record. When you reach this point, you will experience fewer and fewer situations as truly distressing, and you can spend your energy on solving what problems remain and on enjoying yourself in more situations.

CHAPTER 7 SUMMARY

- Column 6 of the Thought Record, "Alternative or Balanced Thoughts," summarizes the important evidence collected and recorded in columns 4 and 5.

- If the evidence in columns 4 and 5 does not support the original hot thought, write in column 6 an alternative view of the situation that is consistent with the evidence.

- If the evidence in columns 4 and 5 only partially supports your original hot thought, write a balanced thought in column 6 that summarizes the evidence both supporting and contradicting your original thought.

- Ask yourself the questions in the Hint Box (p. 95) to help construct an alternative or balanced thought.

- Alternative or balanced thoughts are not merely positive thinking or rationalizations. Instead, they reflect new meanings of situations based on <u>all</u> the available evidence.

- In column 7 of the Thought Record, rerate the intensity of the mood(s) you identified in column 2.

- The shift in emotional response to a situation is often related to the believability of the alternative or balanced thoughts you write.

- If there is no shift in emotional intensity after completing a Thought Record, use the Troubleshooting Guide (p. 102) to discover what else you may need to do to reduce your distress.

- The more Thought Records you complete, the easier it will become to think more flexibly about situations and begin to consider alternative or balanced explanations for events automatically without writing out the evidence.

WORKSHEET 7.2: Complete Thought Record

THOUGHT

1. Situation	2. Moods	3. Automatic Thoughts (Images)
		Answer some or all of the following questions: What was going through my mind just before I started to feel this way? What does this say about me? What does this mean about me? my life? my future? What am I afraid might happen? What is the worst thing that could happen if this is true? What does this mean about how the other person(s) feel(s)/think(s) about me? What does this mean about the other person(s) or people in general? What images or memories do I have in this situation?
Who were you with? What were you doing? When was it? Where were you?	Describe each mood in one word. Rate intensity of mood (0–100%).	

RECORD

4. Evidence That Supports the Hot Thought	5. Evidence That Does Not Support the Hot Thought	6. Alternative/ Balanced Thoughts	7. Rate Moods Now
Circle hot thought in previous column for which you are looking for evidence. Write factual evidence to support this conclusion. (Try to avoid mind-reading and interpretation of facts.)	Ask yourself the questions in the Hint Box (p. 70) to help discover evidence which does not support your hot thought.	Ask yourself the questions in the Hint Box (p. 95) *to* generate alternative or balanced thoughts. Write an alternative or balanced thought. Rate how much you believe in each alternative or balanced thought (0–100%).	Copy the feelings from Column 2. Rerate the intensity of each feeling from 0 to 100% as well as any new records.

Experiments and Action Plans

Michelle enrolled in a Spanish class to prepare for a trip to Mexico. She learned to ask directions, order food, and respond to common conversational questions. When Michelle arrived in Mexico, her taxi driver spoke English, as did the people working in her hotel. After unpacking, Michelle decided to go to the neighborhood pharmacy to buy some post cards and stamps.

In the pharmacy, everyone was speaking Spanish rapidly. Michelle reviewed her language book and then stepped hesitantly up to the counter and spoke the phrases in Spanish she believed would order stamps and post cards. To Michelle's surprise, the woman behind the counter smiled and handed her the number of cards and stamps she wanted to purchase.

Why was Michelle surprised?

Our first learning of something new tends to be intellectual, or "in our head." We know that a particular language is supposed to work in another country, but when we actually speak that language, we doubt it will be understood because the words and phrases are so different from the language most familiar to us. In the beginning, our native language seems the only true way to speak. A new language begins to feel like true communication only after a lot of practice.

Even though Michelle believed that her Spanish phrases were correct, she did not have confidence in the language until she began to receive positive reactions from the people she met in Mexico. As she spoke Spanish more regularly, she gained greater confidence.

Developing alternative and balanced thoughts for your Thought Records may be like writing in a new language for you. Like any new language, these new thoughts probably seem awkward and only partly believable. While your automatic thoughts flow easily like a familiar native language, your alternative thoughts emerge only with great effort. You probably believe the new thoughts "in your head" but they don't feel as if they fit your life experience as well as the old automatic thoughts.

Like Michelle learning Spanish, the best way to increase the believability of your alternative or balanced thoughts is to try them out in your day-to-day life. If these life experiments increase your belief in alternative or balanced thoughts, your improved mood will become more stable. If the experiments do not support your new beliefs, you can use this information to create different alternative thoughts that fit your life experiences better.

BEN'S EXPERIMENT: *Reach out and touch someone.*

Ben's discouraged feelings on Thanksgiving Day were somewhat alleviated by his realization that even though his children and grandchildren didn't need him in the same ways they used to, they still enjoyed his company, asked for his advice, and needed him in different ways. Although recognizing this helped Ben feel better, his new way of thinking was not fully believable to him — even though the evidence seemed to support the new idea. One way for Ben to increase his belief in his new conclusion was to do some "experiments" to test out his alternative thoughts. Ben decided to test out his new conclusions ("They still need me but in different ways and they enjoy being with me"). He called his daughter and son-in-law and offered to help them on a project. His daughter and son-in-law told him that they didn't have any projects to be done. Rather than concluding that he was unwanted, as he had done in the past, Ben decided to carry his experiment further: he asked them if he could help them in any other way.

After thinking for a moment, his daughter told Ben that his granddaughter Amy's best friend had moved out of town. Amy had been feeling lonely, especially after school when she normally played with her friend. Ben eagerly agreed to spend time with Amy two or three times a week after school.

Amy also liked this idea, especially when Ben asked her what she might be interested in doing. She said that she had recently joined a soccer team and would like to practice soccer. Ben agreed to drive her to a field where they would have room to do this. Amy was pleased because the field was too far away to walk or bicycle, and her parents were working and couldn't drive her. Ben was glad to be able to participate in this part of his granddaughter's life.

This experiment led to information that supported Ben's alternative thought ("Even though my children and grandchildren don't need me in the same ways, they still enjoy my company and still ask for my advice"). His family's reaction increased Ben's belief in his new thought, improved his confidence in acting on this belief, and created enjoyable and positive time with Amy. With his previous style of thinking, Ben would have felt rejected and would have given up when his daughter and son-in-law told him that they didn't have any projects ("What's the use? They don't need me any more"). Ben's alternative thoughts gave him the confidence to find new ways to feel needed instead of giving up when his initial offer was declined.

LINDA'S EXPERIMENT: *There is nothing to fear but fear itself.*

Linda's alternative thought, based on the evidence that she had gathered, was that her racing heart and sweating were characteristic of anxiety, not a heart attack. Although her experiences supported the new idea, Linda did not fully believe the new explanation of her symptoms. In order to increase her belief and gather more evidence to support or not support her new understanding, Linda decided to test her thought "I'm not in danger when my heart races and I sweat. These physical changes can be caused by exercise, anxiety, or other factors. I'm not necessarily having a heart attack when I have these experiences."

While sitting in her therapist's office, Linda was convinced that her bodily changes were merely symptoms of anxiety. But in the middle of a panic attack outside her therapist's office, Linda still believed that she was dying of a heart attack when her heart raced and she began to sweat. Simply doing Thought Records was not enough because Linda only fully believed the alternative thoughts when she was not anxious.

Therefore, with her therapist's guidance, Linda began a series of experiments to test her alternative thoughts when she was anxious. First, she and the therapist did a variety of experiments in the office in which she increased her heart rate, and brought on sweating and chest tightness. By running in place or hyperventilating, Linda was able to create within a minute or two all the symptoms that scared her. In the office she was less anxious about these symptoms ("I've brought them on by running or breathing hard") and could see that it was possible to sweat and have a racing heart without having a heart attack.

In a second series of experiments, Linda purposely brought on these symptoms outside the office. On a daily basis, she would raise her heart rate and sweating through exercise and rate her confidence that she was not having a heart attack. If she had thoughts like "I'm OK—but if I exercise any more then I might have a heart attack," she exercised longer, encouraged by her therapist, to test this idea. (Note: Linda had a physical exam before she began exercising strenuously, in which the doctor told her she did not have any heart problems, so it was medically safe for her to keep exercising even though she didn't always think she was safe).

Next, the therapist encouraged Linda to imagine airplane flights from start to finish until she raised her heart rate and sweating through anxiety. These experiments helped convince Linda that anxiety alone could lead to increased heart rate and sweating. During these imaginary flights, Linda became more convinced that the symptoms did not mean she was having a heart attack. Finally, she began scheduling the airplane flights she had been avoiding.

On the way to the airport for the first flight, Linda hoped that her earlier experiments would prevent her from feeling anxious. She was surprised to find that her heart began beating wildly from the moment she left home on the morning of the flight. Linda's heart began racing and she began to sweat. Linda reminded herself of all the times she had felt this way when exercising or anxious and how she had never had a heart attack, even though she thought she would. To test the possibility that the symptoms on the way to the airport were anxiety and not a heart attack, Linda distracted herself from focusing on her body by concentrating on a report she had brought along to write on the trip. After 10 minutes of concentration on the report, she noticed that her heart rate had slowed. Since distraction can reduce anxiety but not a heart attack, Linda began to breathe easier—she was not dying, just anxious.

Over the following months, Linda found it easier to fly. Occasionally she would still become anxious, especially when the plane encountered turbulence. However, she stopped panicking when she gained confidence in the realization that her symptoms indicated anxiety, not a heart attack. Figure 8.1 on page 116 illustrates how Linda planned and charted two of her experiments.

THOUGHT TO BE TESTED		I'm not in danger when my heart races and I sweat. These physical changes can be caused by exercise, anxiety, or other factors. I'm not necessarily having a heart attack when I have these experiences.

Experiment	Prediction	Possible problems	Strategies to overcome these problems	Outcome of experiment	How much does the outcome support the thought that was tested? (0–100%)
In my therapist's office, increase my heart rate by jogging in place.	When I stop jogging, my heart rate will rapidly return to normal.	I may believe that I am having a heart attack and stop the experiment because of that.	I will tell my therapist that I think I am having a heart attack, and my therapist will help me evaluate how to proceed.	My heartbeat increased soon after I began jogging and returned to normal approximately 10 minutes after I stopped jogging.	100%
I will visualize myself in an airport, getting on an airplane and taking off.	My heart rate will increase and I will start to sweat as I am imagining this scene. My heart rate and sweating will return to normal after I stop the visualization.	I may interrupt this experiment if my heart starts to race too fast. I may believe that I am having a heart attack and panic.	If I start to believe that I am having a heart attack, I can come out of the visualization for a minute or two, calm down by doing deep breathing and then restart the visualization and go further with it.	My heart rate increased and I started to sweat the more absorbed I became in this visualization. When I ended the visualization, my heart rate returned to normal and I stopped sweating.	100%

WHAT HAVE I LEARNED FROM THESE EXPERIMENTS?	A rapid heartbeat and sweating can be caused by anxiety or exercise.

FIGURE 8.1. Linda's experiments.

Even after her anxiety became less frequent, Linda continued doing behavioral experiments to strengthen her belief that her symptoms were not dangerous, just uncomfortable. She occasionally let her racing heart continue for 10 or more minutes without distraction to remind herself that a racing heart was not dangerous. Linda knew she had conquered her anxiety when she earned her first "frequent flyer" free airline ticket and was actually happy to be able to schedule another flight—this time for a vacation.

Linda's experiences provide several good guidelines for planning behavioral experiments:

1. Break up experiments into small steps. Small steps are easier to do, and what you learn in each small step can help you make the bigger steps later. Linda began her experiments in her therapist's office by bringing on her symptoms with exercise. Next she used exercise at home to experiment without a therapist present. Finally, she began doing experiments in which her symptoms were brought on by anxiety—first in imagination, then in reality. Her many experiences with a racing heart brought on by exercise (the first small step) helped her cope with a racing heart brought on by anxiety.

2. We usually need to do a number of experiments before we truly believe a new way of thinking about things. Linda believed that her symptoms were not dangerous when she was not anxious. It took a number of experiments and plane flights before she believed her new thought ("A racing heart can be caused by anxiety and is not dangerous") not only when calm but also when anxious. Multiple experiments also helped Linda become skilled at handling her anxiety so that she didn't need to avoid situations in which she anticipated feeling anxious.

3. The whole idea of an experiment is to discover what really happens when we try something new. When experiments don't turn out as we hope, it is time to problem solve, not quit. Because Linda had a surprisingly high degree of anxiety on her first plane flight, she made some changes in her coping plans as she planned for her second trip. First, she drank a glass of milk instead of coffee before leaving for the airport. Second, she left a half hour earlier so that she wouldn't need to rush and would have plenty of time to calm herself if anxious. These two changes reduced two natural causes of increased heart rate (caffeine and rushing). She also took a few minutes for relaxation before leaving the house so her pre-airport heart rate was lower, which made it easier for her to cope with her anxiety.

4 It is helpful to write down your experiments and their outcomes. Writing

down your experiments makes it more likely you will learn from them. When Linda had taken flights before she began her formal experiments, she had just considered herself "lucky" if the flight went well and "a mental case" if she had a panic attack. By writing down her experiments, Linda was able to learn from both her good and bad experiences.

Linda's efforts helped prepare her to cope with her first flight successfully. For her, success did not mean having no anxiety; it meant knowing what to do when she felt anxious. She was also successful because she learned to believe that her rapid heartbeat was caused by anxiety and not a heart attack.

EXERCISE: Doing an Experiment

Look back at the Thought Records you completed at the end of Chapter 6 (Worksheet 6.1) and Chapter 7 (Worksheet 7.2) and choose an alternative or balanced thought that you do not fully believe. Write the alternative or balanced thought on the "Thought to be Tested" lines of Worksheet 8.1. Fill in the columns of the worksheet by designing an experiment that will help you test the alternative or balanced thought. Predict the outcome of the experiment, anticipate possible problems with completing it, and develop strategies to overcome the possible problems. Refer to pages 117–118 for guidelines for planning your experiments.

Do the experiment. Rate the outcome of the experiment and write a summary of what you have learned from the process. If the results of your experiment are not consistent with your alternative or balanced thought, do the experiment again to gather more data, design a different experiment to test your alternative or balanced thought, or develop a different alternative or balanced thought that is consistent with the results of your experiments. There are additional forms for this in the Appendix.

Remember to do experiments in small steps.

Design and carry out several more experiments for the same or different thoughts.

WORKSHEET 8.1: Experiment

THOUGHT TO BE TESTED: _____

_____

_____

Experiment	Prediction	Possible problems	Strategies to overcome these problems	Outcome of experiment	How much does the outcome support the thought that was tested? (0–100%)

WHAT HAVE I LEARNED FROM THESE EXPERIMENTS? _____

_____

_____

_____

VIC'S ACTION PLAN: *The storm before the calm.*

In reading about Ben's and Linda's experiments, you learned how one or more experiments can be done to test out alternative or balanced thoughts developed on the Thought Record. Experiments helped Ben and Linda feel more confident that their alternative beliefs were true.

Sometimes a Thought Record will lead to identification of a problem that needs to be solved. In these cases, you will want to make an action plan after doing the Thought Record.

REMINDER BOX

- If the Thought Record leads to an alternative or balanced thought that fits the data but does not seem believable to you, do a series of behavioral experiments to test out the new beliefs.

- If the Thought Record helps identify a problem to be solved, make an action plan for solving this problem.

Recall Vic's Thought Record in Chapter 7 (Figure 7.1). After reviewing all the evidence, Vic concluded that Judy did care about him and wanted him to stay sober. He rated his belief that Judy cared only 80% because she admitted that she was becoming frustrated with his angry outbursts at home. Vic loved Judy and recognized that he would have to make some changes or he might jeopardize his marriage so he decided to make an action plan.

Vic identified two goals that would improve his marriage. First, he would do more positive things for Judy to show he appreciated her. Second, he would stop having angry outbursts. Working with his therapist, Vic developed the Action Plan in Figure 8.2 to help guide his progress. This worksheet encouraged Vic to be as specific as possible. He had to set a time to begin working on his plan, anticipate problems that could interfere with his success, and create strategies for solving the problems in order to keep moving forward on the action plan. Finally, the worksheet provided a place for Vic to record his progress.

| **GOAL: IMPROVE MY MARRIAGE** | | | | |

Action plan	Time to begin	Possible problems	Strategies to overcome the problems	Progress Report
Do 5 positive things for Judy per day such as kissing, a compliment, helping out, smiling at her, massaging her neck, listening to her complaints without anger, calling from the office to say, "I love you," bringing her coffee.	Today (10/6) when I get home and every morning at 7:30 A.M.	I could be feeling angry with her.	Do the less affectionate things (like helping with the dishes, bringing coffee). Do a Thought Record to see if I can reduce my anger.	10/6—Did 6 positives at night. Felt good. 10/7—Did 5 positives. Judy hugged me for helping. 10/8—Felt angry but did 3 positives anyway. A Thought Record helped.
Stop anger outbursts. Reduce to no more than 3 in the first week, 2 in the second week, 1 in the third week, and no more than once a month after that.	Now	A bad day at work so I arrive home in a bad mood.	Do a Thought Record before leaving the office. Make a plan to handle the work problems before I leave the office. Play good music on the way home. Sit in the driveway and relax until I feel calm enough to enter the house. Tell Judy it was a bad day and that I am trying to stay calm. Ask her to help.	10/6—No problems 10/7—Made a plan to handle a work conflict before I left the office. Arrived home pretty relaxed. 10/8—Played music on the way home. Relaxed for 2 minutes in driveway before going into house. Helped me cope with kids crying without getting angry.
		When I feel angry I explode really quickly.	In conversations with Judy, rate my anger 0–10 every minute when I can see it coming. When my anger gets to a 3, tell Judy I need a break for a few minutes to keep calm. When my anger gets to a 5, take a break and write out a Thought Record. Write out what I hear Judy saying and what I believe to be true. Show Judy this summary to check if we are understanding each other accurately. If I get above a 5 in my anger ratings, tell Judy I need a longer break. Return to the conversation only when my anger is below 3. Take a walk, review my Thought Records, remind myself that Judy loves me, that we have worked out lots of problems in the past, and that we can probably solve this problem, too.	10/6—No anger 10/7—Started to get angry, took a break 3 times and eventually finished the conversation. Judy seemed impressed I was sticking to my plan. 10/8—Only mildly angry. After one break I was OK.

FIGURE 8.2. Vic's Action Plan.

Vic had much greater success in improving his marriage once he made his specific action plans to increase positive interactions with Judy and reduce anger outbursts. He actually used suggestions from the "Strategies to Resolve Problems" column to help him through situations that in previous weeks would have led to anger outbursts. The specific coping plans for handling his anger at different intensities, which he and his therapist developed, were successful in heading off outbursts.

Vic followed this action plan for a number of weeks until he learned to handle most situations without exploding in anger. Whenever he did explode in anger in the following weeks, Vic used these setbacks to identify new problems to be solved and to develop additional, more effective plans for controlling his anger.

MARISSA'S ACTION PLAN: *Light at the end of the tunnel.*

Marissa and her therapist spent several sessions determining the reasons she had become highly suicidal. One of the major reasons Marissa felt so hopeless was that she was convinced she would be fired from her job and not be able to support herself and her children. She had a life insurance policy and thought the accidental death clause would provide for her children until they could support themselves.

On a Thought Record, Marissa tested the automatic thought, "I will be fired." While this thought could not be considered as absolutely true until it happened, Marissa had some pretty convincing evidence that being fired was a real possibility. In the previous month, she had received three warnings from her supervisor—one for chronically arriving at work late in the morning and after lunch and two for "poor work product." In her company, three warnings could be followed by firing.

Marissa felt out of control regarding her job. She was so depressed in the morning that it was hard to get out of bed, even though she knew it would look bad if she were late again. Furthermore, once at work, Marissa had a hard time concentrating on her work so she made errors, leading to poor work in her supervisor's eyes.

Since Marissa's job situation was an immediate problem, she and her therapist soon constructed an action plan to help her solve the problem. They discussed and wrote down a variety of actions Marissa could take to make her job more secure. First, she could tell her supervisor that she was trying to do better and ask for help. This supervisor had complimented Marissa on her work only a few months earlier. Marissa acknowledged that her supervisor might be willing to help if he knew she was trying to do better. Second, Marissa could ask Maggie, a friend in the office whom Marissa trusted, to review her work before Marissa handed it to the supervisor. Finally, Marissa considered a variety of strategies to get herself to work on time even when she was depressed.

Marissa's action strategies led her to be more hopeful about keeping her job. After a few minutes, however, she began to see problems that might interfere. The biggest problem was that she didn't feel comfortable about telling her supervisor she was depressed because she wasn't sure it was safe. Her therapist suggested Marissa think about what she would be willing to say to her supervisor that might enlist his help.

Marissa decided to tell her supervisor that she was under a lot of stress, but that she was working hard to straighten things out so that her job performance was not affected. She thought she could remind her supervisor that her work used to be better and assure him that her current problems were temporary and that she expected her performance to be better soon. Marissa's therapist advised her also to let her supervisor know that she really wanted to keep her job and appreciated his help in letting her know what she needed to do to maintain company quality standards. Marissa's completed Action Plan is shown in Figure 8.3 on page 124.

GOAL: Save My Job

Action plan	Time to begin	Possible problems	Strategies to overcome problems	Progress
Talk to my supervisor about stress, prior positive work history, problems only temporary, want to keep my job, appreciate his help.	Wednesday after group meeting.	Supervisor might be too busy to meet.	Ask him ahead of time for 15-minute meeting.	Tuesday— Supervisor agreed to Wednesday meeting.
		Supervisor might say it's too late to save my job.	Remind him of my positive work earlier in the year. Ask him to reconsider and give me 30 days to improve.	Wednesday—Meeting went pretty well. I cried, which I didn't want to do, but he seemed glad I talked to him and assured me I could have a few more weeks to improve my work .
Ask Maggie to review my work.	Tuesday at lunch.	It will burden our friendship.	I can promise to help Maggie out next summer when she goes on vacation. I can water her houseplants for her.	Maggie agreed to help.
Get to work on time. Set alarm on other side of room so I have to get out of bed. Lay out clothes night before so no decisions to make. Leave 10 minutes early and reward myself with time for cup of coffee at office before I begin.	Tuesday A.M.	I'll go back to bed after alarm goes off.	Make a rule that I have to shower and dress before I "rest a few more minutes."	Tuesday—Arrived on time. Wednesday—Arrived five minutes early. Thursday—Arrived 8 minutes early and enjoyed my coffee.

FIGURE 8.3.   Marissa's Action Plan.

Marissa's hopelessness and thoughts of suicide diminished after she made the Action Plan and began to follow it. Notice that she took several different steps to improve her job prospects. Since her depression was making it difficult for her to function well, she enlisted the help of others for a short time. From her boss, she asked for an appropriate level of help and reminded him of her predepression performance level. She asked her friend Maggie for help and promised to do something for Maggie in return. These steps helped Marissa begin to feel in control again.

EXERCISE: Making an Action Plan

Identify a problem in your life that you would like to change and write your goal on the top line on Worksheet 8.2. Complete the Action Plan, making it as specific as possible. Set a time to begin, identify problems that could interfere with completing your plan, develop strategies for coping with the problems if they should arise, and keep written track of the progress you make. Complete additional Action Plans (which can be found in the Appendix) for other problem areas of your life that you would like to change.

WORKSHEET 8.2: Action Plan

GOAL:_____

Action plan	Time to begin	Possible problems	Strategies to overcome problems	Progress

CHAPTER 8 SUMMARY

- Initially, you may not fully believe your balanced or alternative thoughts.

- Use experiments to test your balanced or alternative thoughts. Experiments can help increase your belief in the new thoughts.

- As your belief in your balanced or alternative thoughts increases, your improved mood will stabilize.

- If the experiments do not support your new beliefs, you can use this information to create different beliefs that reflect your experiences.

- Break experiments into small steps. Small steps are easier to do, and what you learn in each small step can help you make bigger steps later.

- You will usually need to do a number of experiments before you shift old beliefs. For this reason, it is important to keep a written record of experiments in order to track results that accumulate over time.

- Action Plans can help you solve problems that you've identified.

- Action Plans should be specific; they should include coping plans for possible problems, set a time to begin, and record progress made.

CHAPTER 9

Assumptions and Core Beliefs

In many ways, automatic thoughts are similar to flowers and weeds in a garden. Thought Records, experiments, and action plans are tools that enable you to cut the weeds (negative automatic thoughts) at ground level from your garden, making room for the flowers. With practice, these tools will work for you for the rest of your life. Whenever the weeds flourish in your garden, you will know how to work with them. For many people, the skills learned in Chapters 1–8 are sufficient to cope with problems effectively. Other people find that even after using these tools there are still more weeds than flowers, or that every time they get rid of one weed, two others take its place. If you have developed proficiency with Thought Records, Experiments, and Action Plans, and you want deeper changes, then the solution may lie in learning to remove the weeds by their roots.

There are three different levels of belief. Automatic thoughts, with which you have been working up to now are the most accessible and identifiable. Automatic thoughts are the parts of the weeds or flowers that are above ground. Automatic thoughts are rooted beneath the surface in assumptions and core beliefs. The following diagram illustrates the connection between automatic thoughts, assumptions, and core beliefs.

Automatic Thoughts

∧
|

Assumptions

∧
|

Core Beliefs

While automatic thoughts are often stated as verbal messages that we say to ourselves, our assumptions are not as obvious. We frequently must infer them from our actions. If we put our assumptions into words, they can usually be stated as "If . . . then . . . " sentences or "should" statements. For example, one of Marissa's assumptions was "If people get to know me, then they will see how despicable I am and reject and hurt me." One of Vic's assumptions was "I should be the best at everything I do." Related to this belief was a second assumption, "If I do not do things perfectly, then I'm inadequate." Assumptions operate as rules that guide our daily actions and expectations.

The deepest level of cognition is the core belief. Core beliefs are absolutistic statements about ourselves, others, or the world. Marissa's core beliefs included "I'm worthless," "I'm unlovable," and "I'm inadequate." Her core beliefs about others included "Others are dangerous," "People will hurt you," "People are malicious." She believed that the "world was full of insurmountable problems." All of these beliefs are "absolutistic"—there are no qualifications. Marissa does not think, "If I fail, I'm worthless," or, "I'm sometimes worthless"; she believes "I am worthless" (absolutely).

Just as you learned to identify and evaluate your automatic thoughts, you can learn to identify and evaluate your assumptions and core beliefs. Learning to change maladaptive assumptions and core beliefs can help reduce the number of negative, distorted automatic thoughts you have throughout the day. Furthermore, developing new assumptions and core beliefs may reduce your distress and make it easier to change your behavior in ways consistent with your new beliefs. For example, as long as Marissa saw herself as despicable (a core belief), she did not allow people to get to know her. She also behaved in withdrawn and protective ways. If Marissa developed the new core belief "I am likable," she would then be more willing to get close to people. With this new belief, Marissa would more likely be relaxed and show her positive qualities to others.

Where do assumptions and core beliefs come from? Very often we have had them since childhood. Young babies begin to make sense of their world by organizing their experiences into familiar patterns. Very young infants, for example, prefer looking at circles and triangles arranged to resemble a human face than at more randomly arranged geometric shapes.

In the second and third years of life, a child begins to develop language and use it to organize and make sense of experience. Based on experience, a child acquires knowledge, such as "Dogs bite" or "Dogs are friendly" which guides behavior (stay away from or approach an unfamiliar dog). Children also learn rules from other people around them ("Big boys don't cry," "Stoves are hot").

The rules and beliefs a child develops are not necessarily true (e.g., boys and men of all ages do cry), but a young child does not yet have the mental ability to think in more flexible ways. The rules take on anabsolute quality for the child. A 3-year-old girl may believe, "It's bad to hit someone," and be angry with her mother for hitting her brother on the back when he is choking on a piece of food. An older child would be able to see the difference between hitting to hurt and hitting to help.

In most areas of our life we develop more flexible rules and beliefs as we grow older. We learn to approach dogs who are wagging their tails and avoid dogs who are growling. We learn that the same behavior can be "bad" or "good" depending on the context. However, some of our beliefs from childhood stay absolute even into adulthood.

Absolute beliefs may remain fixed if they develop from very traumatic circumstances or if consistent early life experiences convince us that these beliefs are true even as we grow older. For example, Marissa was abused as a child and concluded that she was bad. Even though no child deserves to be abused and adults, not the children, are responsible for the abuse, many abused children come to this conclusion. Why is this so? One possibility is that the explanation that she was bad and being punished for it was less frightening to Marissa as a young child than considering that the adults in her home were out of control or mean. To feel some security as a child, she needed to believe the adults were good.

Vic grew up with an older brother, Doug, who was a star athlete and straight-A student. No matter how well Vic did in school and sports, he was never as successful as Doug. Despite Vic's own successes, he grew up with a core belief that he was inadequate. This belief seemed true to Vic because, in his own mind, no accomplishment was worthwhile unless it was the absolute best (i.e., better than Doug). This belief was supported by the many experiences Vic had growing up listening to parents, teachers, and coaches describe Doug's achievements with pride.

Because core beliefs help us make sense of our world at such a young age, it may never occur to us to evaluate whether they are the most useful ways of understanding our adult experiences. Instead, as adults, we act, think, and feel as if these beliefs are still 100% true.

IDENTIFYING ASSUMPTIONS AND CORE BELIEFS: THE DOWNWARD ARROW TECHNIQUE

One way to identify assumptions and core beliefs is to look for recurring themes in the Thought Records you have completed. If certain types of automatic thoughts repeatedly occur, they may provide a clue to your assumptions and core beliefs.

Vic, after a week-long drinking binge, wanted to better understand what led to his drinking. In evaluating two partially completed Thought Records that preceded his drinking binge and one partially completed Thought Record that he did afterward, Vic noticed themes that connected the three different situations. Vic summarized the three experiences on the Thought Record in Figure 9.1.

THOUGHT RECORD

1. Situation	2. Moods	3. Automatic Thoughts (Images)
Who? What? When? Where?	a. What did you feel? b. Rate each mood (0–100%)	a. What was going though your mind just before you started to feel this way? Any other thoughts? Images? b. Circle the hot thought
1. Received new sales quotas from my manager	Anxious 90%	I won't be able to meet these quotas. I'll fail again.
2. Invited to a family party	Anxious 70%	I'll probably say the wrong thing to my sister.
3. Lying in bed with a hangover	Depressed 95%	I'm just a drunk. I never succeed at anything. I'm hopeless.

FIGURE 9.1. Vic's Thought Record summary.

Do you notice any theme in the way Vic thinks about himself that might suggest a

core belief? _____

The themes that appear in Vic's automatic thoughts appear to be failure and inadequacy. Vic seems to have core beliefs such as, "I'm a failure," "I'm not good enough," or "I can't handle things."

A second way to identify core beliefs is called the **downward arrow technique**. This is essentially the method you learned in Chapter 5, where you learned to ask questions such as, "What does this situation mean about me?" to identify your automatic thoughts present in a situation (refer to the box on page 51). Once you identify automatic thoughts, you can ask yourself the same or similar questions to help identify underlying assumptions and core beliefs. For example, for any given automatic thought you can ask yourself, "If this were true, what would be so bad about that? What does this mean about me?"

Sometimes repeatedly asking yourself "What does this mean about me?" will help reveal core beliefs about yourself that underlie automatic thoughts previously identified.

For example, if you had the automatic thought, "I don't think Marsha likes me," and this thought contributed to depressed feelings, the downward arrow technique would help you find the underlying belief in this way:

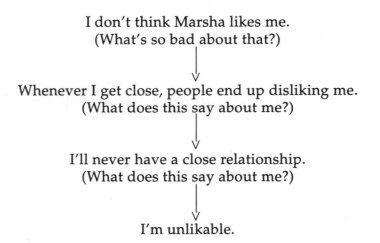

I don't think Marsha likes me.
(What's so bad about that?)

↓

Whenever I get close, people end up disliking me.
(What does this say about me?)

↓

I'll never have a close relationship.
(What does this say about me?)

↓

I'm unlikable.

In this example of the downward arrow technique, the automatic thought ("I don't think Marsha likes me") is about a particular situation. When we identify the core belief related to the feelings of depression ("I'm unlikable"), it is an absolute statement that seems unchangeable.

The preceding examples illustrate how to identify assumptions and core beliefs about one's self. We also have assumptions and core beliefs about others and the world. The downward arrow technique can be used to identify beliefs about others or the world by modifying the questions. For example, beliefs about other people can be identified with the downward arrow technique by asking, "What does this situation mean or say about other people?" Assumptions or core beliefs about the world can be identified by asking questions like "What does this situation say or mean about the world and how it operates?" Examples of using the downward arrow technique to identify core beliefs about others and the world follow:

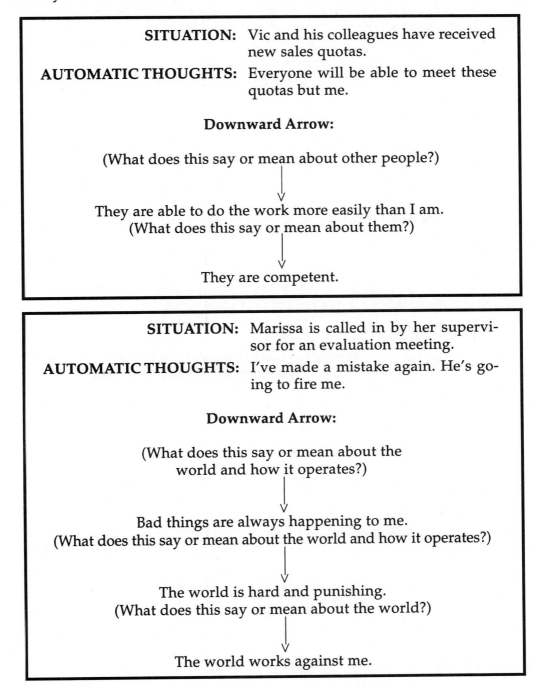

SITUATION: Vic and his colleagues have received new sales quotas.

AUTOMATIC THOUGHTS: Everyone will be able to meet these quotas but me.

Downward Arrow:

(What does this say or mean about other people?)

They are able to do the work more easily than I am.
(What does this say or mean about them?)

They are competent.

SITUATION: Marissa is called in by her supervisor for an evaluation meeting.

AUTOMATIC THOUGHTS: I've made a mistake again. He's going to fire me.

Downward Arrow:

(What does this say or mean about the world and how it operates?)

Bad things are always happening to me.
(What does this say or mean about the world and how it operates?)

The world is hard and punishing.
(What does this say or mean about the world?)

The world works against me.

Sometimes identifying core beliefs about the self will be enough to understand a recurrent problem in your life. Often, however, core beliefs about the self tell only part of the story. Identifying core beliefs about others and the world can complete our understanding of why a situation is so distressing. For example, Vic would have been less concerned about failing to meet the sales quota if he had thought others would fail, too. Seeing others as competent intensified his distress and added to his perception of himself as inadequate.

Marissa's core belief that the "world is hard and punishing and works against her" certainly adds to her depression and hopelessness. She had difficulty putting forth effort day after day because of her belief that eventually the world would crash down on her despite her best efforts. In fact, it was a testimony to Marissa's courage that she continued to work hard in her life despite her beliefs about the world.

Negative beliefs about the world are more common for people who have witnessed or experienced trauma; experienced harsh economic conditions without relief; lived in chaotic, unpredictable circumstances; been hurt by persistent discrimination; or lived through life experiences of any kind that were persistently harmful or unpredictably punishing. Children who have these types of experiences seem particularly vulnerable to developing negative core beliefs about the world, but powerful negative experiences can help create negative core beliefs at any age.

Similarly, negative core beliefs about others usually develop from traumatic or persistently negative interactions with other people. Sometimes, as we saw with Vic, an indirect experience such as observing a highly successful sibling can help create a view of others that causes distress. Vic's positive view of others ("They are competent") linked with his negative core belief about himself ("I'm inadequate") helps explain the level of his anxiety and apprehension.

Several exercises follow (Worksheets 9.1, 9.2, 9.3, and 9.4) to help you discover some of your negative core beliefs. See if you can uncover core beliefs about yourself, others, and the world. If you have difficulty identifying a negative core belief in one of these areas, it may mean that you don't have this type of negative core belief or that the Thought Record you have chosen does not involve this type of negative core belief. In any case, if you can identify even one core belief, continue with the rest of this chapter.

EXERCISE: Identifying Cognitive Themes

Referring to the Thought Records you completed in Chapter 6 (Worksheet 6.1) and Chapter 7 (Worksheet 7.2), try to identify themes that connect two or more Thought Records. Look particularly for similarities in column 3, Automatic Thoughts, of numerous Thought Records. Summarize the different thoughts by completing the sentences on Worksheet 9.1.

WORKSHEET 9.1: Identifying Cognitive Themes

1. I am_____

_____

2. Others are_____

_____

3. The world is_____

_____

EXERCISE: Identifying Core Beliefs About Self

Refer again to the Thought Records you completed in Chapter 6 (Worksheet 6.1) and Chapter 7 (Worksheet 7.2). Pick one Thought Record on which you recorded intense moods. Complete Worksheet 9.2 based on that Thought Record. End the exercise when you arrive at an absolute statement about yourself. You may have to continue to ask yourself the question "What does this say or mean about me?" more times than printed on the worksheet or you may arrive at a core belief after asking the question one or two times.

WORKSHEET 9.2: Downward Arrow Technique:
Identifying Core Beliefs About Self

Situation (from Thought Record)

_____

_____

What does this say or mean about me?

↓

_____

What does this say or mean about me?

↓

_____

What does this say or mean about me?

↓

_____

What does this say or mean about me?

↓

_____

EXERCISE: Identifying Core Beliefs About Others

Pick one Thought Record on which you recorded intense mood. Complete Worksheet 9.3 based on that Thought Record. End the exercise when you arrive at an absolute statement about other people. You may have to continue to ask yourself the question "What does this say or mean about other people?" more times than printed on the worksheet or you may arrive at a core belief after asking the question one or two times.

**WORKSHEET 9.3.   Downward Arrow Technique:
Identifying Core Beliefs About Others**

Situation (from Thought Record)

_____

_____

What does this say or mean about other people?

↓

_____

What does this say or mean about other people?

↓

_____

What does this say or mean about other people?

↓

_____

What does this say or mean about other people?

↓

_____

EXERCISE: Identifying Core Beliefs About the World

Pick one Thought Record on which you recorded intense mood. Complete Worksheet 9.4 based on that Thought Record. End the exercise when you arrive at an absolute statement about the world. You may have to continue to ask yourself the question "What does this say or mean about the world?" more times than printed on the worksheet or you may arrive at a core belief after asking the question one or two times.

WORKSHEET 9.4. Downward Arrow Technique: Identifying Core Beliefs About the World

Situation (from Thought Record)

_____

_____

What does this say or mean about the world?

↓

_____

What does this say or mean about the world?

↓

_____

What does this say or mean about the world?

↓

_____

What does this say or mean about the world?

↓

_____

Whatever the origins of the core beliefs that contribute to your distress, this section and the next teach you methods for changing them. For Marissa, a change in core beliefs meant learning to see that the world is not always hard and punishing and that sometimes things go her way. A belief that things can sometimes go her way encouraged Marissa to begin to look for relationships and environments that she could count on to be more consistently supportive. She then learned to use these supports to help her cope with the harsher relationships and environments in her life. For Vic, a change in core beliefs meant learning to feel good even when he was not "the best." Vic also benefited from learning to see a middle ground between "the best" and "complete failure."

TESTING CORE BELIEFS

Core beliefs can take longer to change than automatic thoughts because we require a lot more evidence over time to convince us that these absolute and usually long-held beliefs are not 100% true. Fortunately, you have already learned a lot about testing out your thoughts, so you already have some tools to begin testing core beliefs. Unlike previous chapters, you will do most of the following exercises in this chapter over weeks or months instead of hours or days to accommodate the longer time frame necessary for changing core beliefs.

Just as you tested automatic thoughts, you can test a belief like, "I'm unlovable" by listing evidence that supports and does not support the belief. Be careful: it is easy to miss facts that don't fit our expectations and thus ignore evidence which contradicts our negative beliefs.

Marissa, for example, believed that she was unlovable. When she first tested this idea, she did not count evidence like invitations to lunch from people at work, warm greetings from several of the other secretaries when she arrives at work, the love of her children, the love of some friends—even when they told her. This was important evidence that Marissa was lovable, but Marissa didn't count it because she thought, "They were just feeling sorry for me," or "They don't really know me yet."

HELPFUL HINTS

☞

> Keep track of *all* the evidence that might disagree with your negative core belief, even if it seems small or unimportant to you.

Be certain to notice and remember all the little things that suggest that your negative core belief is not 100% true. Noticing small positive experiences is particularly important to counteract an automatic tendency to remember the small negative experiences that support our core beliefs. By actively looking for small experiences that contradict our negative core belief, we ensure a better balance to our views.

In order to fully evaluate a core belief, you may need to record evidence that disagrees with this belief for weeks or even months. Since the belief has probably been with you for years, you may need a lot of data to convince yourself that the belief is not 100% true.

EXERCISE: Recording Evidence That a Core Belief Is Not 100% True

Choose a core belief you would like to evaluate. On Worksheet 9.5 start recording experiences that show that the belief is not 100% true all the time. Try to find one piece of evidence every day the first week. Even very small experiences count. You'll have to look really hard, because you are probably not used to seeing the good things about this area of your life.

Once you can find a piece of evidence nearly every day, try looking for two or three bits of evidence every day. Don't worry if the things you write down seem trivial or if you are unsure that they are really true. After several weeks, when you have 20 or 25 items on your list, you can look at them all and draw an overall conclusion about whether your original negative core belief accurately describes your whole experience.

HELPFUL HINTS

This chapter introduces you to a variety of exercises which can help you change the core beliefs which lead to unhappiness or distress in your life. Unlike earlier chapters, most of the worksheets (9.5–9.9) described here require you to keep records for weeks or months to gather enough evidence to evaluate your old and new beliefs. Don't expect to do all the worksheets in this section simultaneously. Work on one worksheet for a while, write down what you learn, and then move to another one.

WORKSHEET 9.5.   Core Belief Record: Recording Evidence That a Core Belief Is Not 100% True

Core Belief: _____

Evidence or experiences that suggest that the core belief is not 100% true all the time:

1. _____
2. _____
3. _____
4. _____
5. _____
6. _____
7. _____
8. _____
9. _____
10. _____
11. _____
12. _____
13. _____
14. _____
15. _____
16. _____
17. _____
18. _____
19. _____
20. _____
21. _____
22. _____
23. _____
24. _____
25. _____

While you are keeping track of evidence that your core belief does not always fit your experiences, you can also test the belief with experiments. With Marissa's belief, "I'm unlovable," she predicted that if she tried to be friends with people, they would reject her. As you learned to do in Chapter 8, Marissa wrote down her experiments so that she could see the whole picture and learn from the results. Her record of experiments is shown in Figure 9.2.

Experiment	Prediction from my negative core belief	What actually happened
Smile at 10 people.	All will look away.	2 looked away. 6 smiled back. 2 said hello.
Ask Julio to have breakfast.	He'll say no.	He said yes, if we could eat by 9:00 A.M.
Invite someone to the movies.	The person will say no.	First two people had other plans this weekend. Third person said yes.

FIGURE 9.2. Marissa's experiments regarding lovability.

After you have kept a prediction record like Marissa's for a number of experiments, you can look it over and see if it supports your negative belief. Do you think Marissa's experiments provide evidence that she is unlovable?

Marissa's experiments do not prove that Marissa is unlovable as she expected they would. Some of the people in her life seem to be responding positively to her. Of course, Marissa needs to do more experiments to see if people continue to respond positively as they get to know her better. It is important to do a number of experiments before drawing conclusions.

Sometimes your experiments may turn out as negatively as you predict. For example, suppose Marissa had been rejected by everyone—no one smiled, Julio said no to breakfast, and no one agreed to go to the movies. Does this mean she is unlovable? Maybe yes, maybe no. This would be a good time for Marissa to talk with friends or a counselor to find out if she is doing something to keep people away. One man who did this found out that he was always being told no because he invited people to do things too late (e.g., he would call people Saturday morning to do things Saturday night).

Once you've done a number of experiments, it can be helpful to look over your results and write out a new belief that describes your experiences more accurately than the old belief. For Marissa, her new belief might be "I'm likable to some people." Can you see how this is a more accurate belief for her than "I'm unlovable?"

IDENTIFYING AND STRENGTHENING ALTERNATIVE CORE BELIEFS

As you identify and test your negative core beliefs, you may identify alternative beliefs that are less absolute and negative. Marissa experimented with the beliefs, "Some people love me" and "I can learn to do things, even if they seem hard." Vic came to believe, "It's OK to make mistakes—that's how we learn." Once you identify new core beliefs, keep looking for evidence to support them because it will take some time before they are as strong as your old negative beliefs.

If you have not already done so, develop an alternative core belief that can help explain the observations you recorded on Worksheet 9.5 that don't fit your negative core belief. Labeling these experiences with a new core belief is like setting up a new file in your mind. In the same way that a well-organized filing system at home or work helps you store and retrieve information, a newly labeled core belief helps you store and remember experiences by giving you a place in which to organize them. Without the new file, experiences that don't fit the negative core belief would be either misfiled or simply discarded. The new alternative core belief provides a name under which you can remember *all* the experiences you have, not just the negative ones.

To identify a possible new core belief, examine the information you gathered on Worksheet 9.5. What is an alternative core belief that could explain these experiences? Sometimes the alternative core belief is the opposite of the initial core belief. For example, Marissa shifted her belief from "I'm unlovable" to "I'm lovable." This new belief did not mean that she expected everyone to love her; it simply meant that some people found her lovable. At other times, the alternative core belief may change an absolute belief to a qualified belief. For example, Marissa shifted her belief, "People will hurt you" to "Some people may be hurtful while others are kind and giving." At still other times, the alternative core belief may evaluate experience from a completely new perspective. For example, Vic shifted his belief that his success and worth hinged on being the best to a belief that he was worthwhile as long as he maintained a mutually satisfying relationship with his wife and children.

EXERCISE: Recording Evidence That Supports an Alternative Core Belief

At the top of Worksheet 9.6 write out an alternative core belief that explains the experiences you recorded on Worksheet 9.5. Then begin recording small events and experiences that support the new core belief. Over the next few months, continue to write down experiences that support your new belief.

WORKSHEET 9.6. **Core Belief Record: Recording Evidence That Supports an Alternative Core Belief**

New Core Belief: _____

Evidence or experiences that support the new belief:

1. _____
2. _____
3. _____
4. _____
5. _____
6. _____
7. _____
8. _____
9. _____
10. _____
11. _____
12. _____
13. _____
14. _____
15. _____
16. _____
17. _____
18. _____
19. _____
20. _____
21. _____
22. _____
23. _____
24. _____
25. _____

To keep track of how your beliefs are changing, it is helpful to rate the strength of your new belief on a scale similar to the one you used in Chapter 3 to rate your moods. For example, when Marissa started looking at the belief that she was unlovable, she believed it completely, so her lovability scale looked like this:

I'm Lovable

X

| 0% | 25% | 50% | 75% | 100% |

After keeping her new Core Belief Record (Worksheet 9.6) for 10 weeks, Marissa's scale looked like this:

I'm Lovable

X

| 0% | 25% | 50% | 75% | 100% |

While this may look like a small change to you, it was very important to Marissa. This was the first time in her life that she had felt at all lovable. This much belief in her lovability allowed her to begin really feeling loved by her children and friends. She kept track of small signs of lovability for a year and her rating eventually reached 70%.

EXERCISE: Rating Confidence in New Core Beliefs Over Time

On the first line of Worksheet 9.7, write the new core belief you developed for Worksheet 9.6. Then enter the date and rate the new core belief by placing an "X" on the scale above the number that best matches how much you think this new belief is true. To measure your progress in strengthening your new core belief, rerate the new core belief every few weeks.

WORKSHEET 9.7: Rating Confidence in a New Core Belief

New core belief: _____

Ratings of confidence in the belief

Date: _____

| 0 | 25 | 50 | 75 | 100 |

Date: _____

| 0 | 25 | 50 | 75 | 100 |

Date: _____

| 0 | 25 | 50 | 75 | 100 |

Date: _____

| 0 | 25 | 50 | 75 | 100 |

Date: _____

| 0 | 25 | 50 | 75 | 100 |

Date: _____

| 0 | 25 | 50 | 75 | 100 |

Date: _____

| 0 | 25 | 50 | 75 | 100 |

Date: _____

| 0 | 25 | 50 | 75 | 100 |

As you record more experiences on Worksheet 9.6 and do the remaining exercises in this chapter, your new core belief should become more believable to you. Confidence in a new core belief usually takes months to develop, so don't be discouraged if your confidence rating increases at a very slow pace—or even remains in one spot for a long time. The more experiences you notice and write down to support the new belief, the more likely it is that you will begin to have confidence that the new belief has merit.

It is not necessary to be 100% confident of your new core belief. In fact, most people begin to feel better when their confidence in the new belief reaches midpoint on the scale. Rating yourself on a scale helps you give yourself credit for partial success and for progress.

Vic learned to use rating scales to reduce his perfectionism. For example, his therapist taught Vic to rate his anger at work and at home on an "anger control" scale. The following scale shows how Vic rated his anger control in a conversation with Judy.

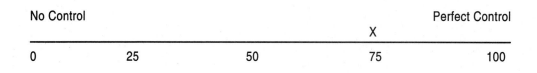

No Control			X	Perfect Control
0	25	50	75	100

In the conversation, Vic became irritated and raised his voice several times. He even pounded the table with his fist once. But he did not criticize Judy or leave the house or behave in any way she considered threatening. He stayed on topic and took one 3-minute break to cool down when his anger started to feel out of control.

Before learning to rate his experiences, Vic would have judged the conversation as an anger control "failure" because he was not perfectly in control all the time. Evaluating this experience as a "failure" would have discouraged Vic and perhaps added to his hopelessness about learning to control his anger. Using the scale shifted Vic's perspective. He was able to see that he was not a failure: he was 75% successful instead of 0% successful. Even though he was very angry, he did not explode or hurt Judy. For these reasons, he and Judy considered his efforts worthwhile, even though he showed less than perfect control. Recognizing his partial success showed Vic that he was making progress and helped him feel good about what he was doing well.

Rating your experiences on a scale may be equally helpful in your life. If you have changes you are trying to make or experiences that you tend to discount or see as "failures" if they are not perfect, try rating them on a scale.

See what difference it makes if you focus on the partial positive of the experience instead of looking solely at the negative.

REMINDER BOX

Use a scale to rate experiences you tend to see in "all" or "nothing" or "success" or "failure" terms. Also use a scale to track progress in changing a behavior or mood. Notice how it feels to look at the positive portion of the scale. Try to give yourself credit for any progress represented on the scale.

EXERCISE: Rating Experiences

On Worksheet 9.8 rate experiences you tend to evaluate in "all" or "nothing" terms. For each scale, describe the situation and write what quality you will rate. Notice how it feels to give yourself partial credit instead of evaluating yourself in "all" or "nothing" terms. (The Appendix provides an additional worksheet that you can copy to rate more experiences.) After you have rated several experiences on these scales, summarize what you learn at the bottom of Worksheet 9.8. For example, Vic wrote, "Even partial successes are worthwhile."

WORKSHEET 9.8. Rating Personal Experiences

Situation:_____ Quality I am rating:_____

0	25	50	75	100

Situation:_____ Quality I am rating:_____

0	25	50	75	100

Situation:_____ Quality I am rating:_____

0	25	50	75	100

Situation:_____ Quality I am rating:_____

0	25	50	75	100

Situation:_____ Quality I am rating:_____

0	25	50	75	100

Situation:_____ Quality I am rating:_____

0	25	50	75	100

Summary:_____

_____

_____

_____

_____

An additional method to evaluate and strengthen new core beliefs is reviewing your past for experiences that support the new belief. In this method, you remember and write down experiences you had in the past that are consistent with your new belief. You may have to think for a long time or talk to other people who knew you at different stages of your life to remember this information. Marissa decided to do the historical test with her new core belief, "I am lovable" (Figure 9.3). Note that Marissa summarized her history in relationship to her new core belief at the bottom of the worksheet.

NEW CORE BELIEF TO BE TESTED: *I am lovable*

Age	Experiences I had that are consistent with the new core belief
Birth–2	In pictures I look lovable. Aunt Rose tells me that I was adorable and that my grandmother affectionately called me "Love Queen."
3–5	Our neighbors always told my mother that I could stay with them any time. They even said they would adopt me, although I think they were joking. I developed a strong relationship with my first teacher. I think she truly liked me.
6–12	My dog always seemed sad when I went to school and greeted me with affection when I came home. Teachers were nice to me. My girl scout troop leader went out of her way to drive me to meetings.
13–18	I had my first boyfriend. I'm not sure why he liked me, but apparently he was attracted to me. We got married. I had my first baby, and as difficult as those first few years were, the baby loved me.
19–25	My second child was born. He also loved and loves me. I was married a second time.
26–35	I decided that I deserved more than I was getting from my marriage. I had the strength to leave. I received support from people who cared about me.
36–40	My children tell me that they love me and that I've done a good job as a parent. I have two good friends who have been close to me for three years. Some people at work ask me to go to lunch with them. Some friends tell me they love me. **SUMMARY:** I seem to be lovable to some people even though others have hurt me. At every point in my life at least one person has liked me or loved me.

FIGURE 9.3. Marissa's historical test of the new core belief.

Because the experiences Marissa recorded were inconsistent with her old core belief, "I'm unlovable," Marissa had difficulty remembering them. In doing the exercise, Marissa relied on relatives and conversations with her therapist to retrieve some of the information. Marissa found it helpful to review her historical test and add to it as she remembered other experiences that were consistent with her new belief.

EXERCISE: Historical Test of New Core Belief

To strengthen one of your new core beliefs, review your life history looking for evidence that is consistent with this new belief. Write the evidence on Worksheet 9.9. When you have recorded experiences for each age period, write a summary describing how this information supports your new core beliefs.

WORKSHEET 9-9: Historical Test of New Core Belief

NEW CORE BELIEF: _____

Age	Experiences I had that are consistent with the new core belief
Birth–2	
3–5	
6–12	
13–18	
19–25	
26–35	
36–50	
51–65	
66+	

SUMMARY:

_____

_____

_____

The learning experiences in this chapter plant the seeds for new core beliefs. These new core beliefs will help you begin to feel happier and, as they become stronger, you will have fewer negative automatic thoughts. However, there will still be times in your life when you feel greater levels of depression, anxiety, anger, or other distressing moods. There will still be life events that are difficult to face. You may have illnesses or other physical experiences that affect your moods, behaviors, and thoughts. During times of distress, you can expect that negative thoughts and negative core beliefs will return. At those times, it will be helpful to review the evidence you have gathered and written in Thought Records, Experiments, Action Plans, Core Belief Records and Ratings, and Historical Tests of Core Beliefs. Keeping and reviewing these records can reinforce new beliefs until they are present in even the most difficult circumstances.

CHAPTER 9 SUMMARY

- Assumptions and core beliefs are the roots of our automatic thoughts.

- Assumptions can be stated in "If . . . then . . . " terms, while core beliefs are absolutistic statements.

- Maladaptive assumptions and beliefs can be weakened at the same time new assumptions are identified and strengthened.

- Core beliefs can be identified by looking for themes in Thought Records and/or with the downward arrow technique.

- Core beliefs may be about oneself, others, or the world.

- Core beliefs can be tested by looking for evidence that they are true or not 100% true.

- New core beliefs can be strengthened by recording experiences that are consistent with the new belief, rating your confidence in your new belief, conducting experiments to test the new belief, and doing a historical test of the new belief.

- Core beliefs often shift gradually, but over time they become stronger and more stable and exert a powerful influence over the way you think, behave, and feel.

CHAPTER 10

Understanding Depression

Although emotions generally enrich our lives, too much emotion can be disruptive. While all the chapters of this book teach general skills for managing moods, the final three chapters provide specialized information that can help you reduce the frequency and severity of five moods that create distress for people: depression, anxiety, anger, guilt, and shame. You can read only those chapters that describe the moods you would like to understand and change.

In *Mind Over Mood*, you learn about depression through the lives of Ben, Vic, and Marissa. Ben's depression was rather recent and followed important life changes. Vic, in addition to alcoholism, had been struggling for most of his life with low self-esteem and a sense of worthlessness. Marissa's depression symptoms included suicide attempts, low self-esteem and feelings of guilt. Depression includes not only sad mood but also numerous cognitive, behavioral, physical and emotional symptoms. When these symptoms are severe, chronic, or occur repeatedly, they may interfere with our personal relationships or our work.

EXERCISE: Identifying and Assessing Symptoms of Depression

To help identify the symptoms of depression you are experiencing, rate the symptoms listed on the *Mind Over Mood* Depression Inventory on Worksheet 10.1. Fill out this inventory periodically as you use this book to assess how your depression is changing and which interventions are most worthwhile.

Score the inventory by adding up the numbers you circled for all the items. For example, if you circled 3 for each item, your score would be 57 (3 X 19 items). If you couldn't decide between two numbers for an item and circled both, add only the higher number. Compare your scores once or twice each week to see if your symptoms are decreasing and which symptoms are improving and which are not.

To chart change, record your *Mind Over Mood* Depression Inventory scores on Worksheet 10.2 on page 156. Mark each column with the date you completed the Depression Inventory. Then put an X in the column across from your score.

You may find that your scores fluctuate from week to week or do not improve each and every time you fill out the inventory. Some weeks your score may be higher (more depressed) than the week before. This is not unusual nor is it a bad sign; in fact, it reflects a pattern of recovery. Decreasing scores over time are a sign that the changes you are making are contributing to your improvement.

You may have noted that the symptoms on the *Mind Over Mood* Depression Inventory are cognitive, behavioral, emotional, and physical changes, just as in the model for understanding problems described in Chapter 1. Cognitive symptoms of depression include self-criticism, hopelessness, suicidal thoughts, concentration difficulties, and overall negativity. Behavior changes associated with depression include withdrawal from other people, not doing as many activities that are enjoyable or pleasurable, and having difficulty "getting started" with activities. Physical symptoms associated with depression include insomnia, sleeping more or less than usual, being tired, eating less or more, and weight changes. The emotional symptoms that accompany depression include feelings of sadness, irritability, anger, guilt, and nervousness.

Does it surprise you to learn that some of these symptoms are characteristic of depression? Some people believe that problems with sleep, appetite, motivation, or anger are separate from and in addition to depression. But for most people, these symptoms are associated with depression, and successful treatment of depression results in improvement in all the associated symptoms.

WORKSHEET 10.1: *Mind Over Mood* **Depression Inventory**

Circle one number for each item that best describes how much you have experienced each symptom over the last week.

	Not at all	Sometimes	Frequently	Most of the time
1. Sad or depressed mood	0	1	2	3
2. Feeling guilty	0	1	2	3
3. Irritable mood	0	1	2	3
4. Less interest or pleasure in usual activities	0	1	2	3
5. Withdraw from or avoid people	0	1	2	3
6. Find it harder than usual to do things	0	1	2	3
7. See myself as worthless	0	1	2	3
8. Trouble concentrating	0	1	2	3
9. Difficulty making decisions	0	1	2	3
10. Suicidal thoughts	0	1	2	3
11. Recurrent thoughts of death	0	1	2	3
12. Spend time thinking about a suicide plan	0	1	2	3
13. Low self-esteem	0	1	2	3
14. See the future as hopeless	0	1	2	3
15. Self-critical thoughts	0	1	2	3
16. Tiredness or loss of energy	0	1	2	3
17. Significant weight loss or decrease in appetite (do not include weight loss from a diet plan)	0	1	2	3
18. Change in sleep pattern—difficulty sleeping or sleeping more or less than usual	0	1	2	3
19. Decreased sexual desire	0	1	2	3

Score (of total circled numbers)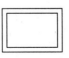

WORKSHEET 10.2: *Mind over Mood Depression Inventory Scores*

Score																		
57																		
54																		
51																		
48																		
45																		
42																		
39																		
36																		
33																		
30																		
27																		
24																		
21																		
18																		
15																		
12																		
9																		
6																		
3																		
0																		
Date																		

COGNITIVE ASPECTS OF DEPRESSION

Aaron T. Beck has pioneered our modern understanding of depression. In the 1960s, Beck demonstrated that depression was characterized by thought patterns that actually maintained the depressed mood. For example, Beck noted that when we are depressed we have negative thoughts about self (self-criticism), about the world (general negativity), and about our future (hopelessness). The following sections describe these three aspects of depressed thinking in detail.

Negative Thoughts About Self

Before Marissa began cognitive therapy, she was extremely self-critical. For example, she thought, "I must be worthless for all these awful things to have happened to me," "I'm no good as a mother or as a person," "If I were a good person, I wouldn't have been sexually abused," "On some level, I probably deserved to be beaten by my husbands." The core belief underlying each of these thoughts is, "I'm worthless" or "I'm no good."

Almost everyone who is depressed thinks these types of self-critical thoughts. The thoughts are damaging because they contribute to low self-esteem, low self-confidence, and relationship problems, and they can interfere with our willingness to do things to help us feel better.

To demonstrate how self-criticism plays a role in your life, remember a time when your self-esteem or self-confidence was particularly low. It may have been a time when you felt worthless and unlovable. Picture in your mind the moment you were feeling most depressed and remember or speculate what you may have been thinking. Did you have any negative thoughts about yourself? If so, write them here:

_____

_____

_____

_____

_____

These thoughts illustrate the self-critical thoughts associated with depression.

Negative Thoughts About the World

Thinking about your current experiences in a negative way is another characteristic of depressive thinking. We often do not take events at face value: We interpret or misinterpret events that occur around us. An example of this is "reading between the lines" when a friend, relative, or coworker is talking. When we are depressed we often perceive others as negative, mean, or critical.

Negative thinking about the world is a style of thinking in which we notice and remember negative aspects of our experiences more vividly than positive or neutral events. For example, when we are depressed we tend to look at and remember the articles in the newspaper that report disasters and not remember the articles that report positive events. Focusing on the two out of ten chores that did not get done on a Saturday would be another example of negative thinking about the world.

Negative Thoughts About the Future

During his first therapy session, Ben's hopelessness was revealed in his statement, "What's the use? The rest of my life will be filled with illness and death." After his wife's successful battle with cancer and the death of his good friend Louie, Ben had come to believe that his own life and the lives of people he was close to would be one tragedy after another, culminating eventually in his own death. He was unable to envision anything other than a bleak future.

When we are depressed we imagine that the future will be completely negative. This prediction or anticipation that events will turn out negatively is called hopelessness. Examples of this type of thinking include "I'll blow it," "Nobody there will like me," "I won't be good at it." A negative attitude toward the future may also manifest itself in thoughts like, "I'll never get out of this depression" or "What's the use in trying? I'll never get any better." We may anticipate that a conversation will go poorly, a new relationship won't work out, a problem can't be solved, or that there is no way out of the depression. In its most extreme form, hopelessness can contribute to thoughts of suicide.

To demonstrate how negative thinking about the future functions in your life, identify an activity you sometimes enjoy but do not do when you are depressed because you predict it will not turn out well. Write in the space at the top of the next page the activity you avoid and your negative prediction of how it will turn out.

_____

_____

_____

_____

_____

_____

EXERCISE: Identifying Cognitive Aspects of Depression

Worksheet 10.3 lists some negative thoughts that people frequently have when they are depressed. To see if you've had these types of negative thoughts and to help you distinguish among them, check each thought you have had and indicate whether each thought is negative toward self, the future, or the world.

WORKSHEET 10.3: Identifying Cognitive Aspects of Depression

Check each thought you have had		Is the thought negative toward self, future, or world
_____	1. I'm no good.	_____
_____	2. I'm a failure.	_____
_____	3. Nobody likes me.	_____
_____	4. Things will never get better.	_____
_____	5. I'm a loser.	_____
_____	6. I'm worthless.	_____
_____	7. No one can help me.	_____
_____	8. I've let people down.	_____
_____	9. Others are better than I am.	_____
_____	10. (S)he hates me.	_____
_____	11. I messed up again.	_____
_____	12. My life is a disaster.	_____
_____	13. (S)he dislikes me.	_____
_____	14. I'm hopeless.	_____
_____	15. Others are disappointed in me.	_____
_____	16. I can't change.	_____

Following are the answers to Worksheet 10.3. Review the pertinent sections of this chapter to clarify any differences between your answers and the ones given.

ANSWERS to Worksheet 10.3

1. I'm no good. .... self
2. I'm a failure. .... self
3. Nobody likes me. .... self/world
4. Things will never get better. .... future
5. I'm a loser. .... self
6. I'm worthless. .... self
7. No one can help me. .... world/future
8. I've let people down. .... self
9. Others are better than I am. .... world
10. (S)he hates me. .... world
11. I messed up again. .... self
12. My life is a disaster. .... self
13. (S)he dislikes me. .... world
14. I'm hopeless. .... future/self
15. Others are disappointed in me. .... world
16. I can't change. .... self

TREATMENT FOR DEPRESSION

Depression can almost always be helped. All the techniques taught in this book were originally developed to help people overcome depression. This section summarizes the treatment approaches that have been shown to be most effective in reducing depression: cognitive restructuring, medication, improving interpersonal relationships, and activity scheduling. Although cognitive restructuring may be most important to long-term reduction of depression, treatment often begins with activity scheduling and/or medication.

Cognitive Restructuring

Depressed people tend to notice and remember negative aspects of their experiences more readily than positive or neutral aspects. They also are more likely to interpret their lives with a negative bias, while nondepressed people interpret events with a positive bias.

The central goal of cognitive therapy for depression is to teach people how to test negative thoughts by reviewing all the information in their lives—positive and neutral as well as negative. Chapters 4-7 taught you how to evaluate your negative thoughts and learn to think in more adaptive ways to reduce your depression. This process is called cognitive restructuring.

Medication

If you experience intense depression or long-lasting depression, or if your depression includes physiological symptoms, such as disruption in sleep, jitteriness, fatigue, or loss of appetite, your therapist is likely to recommend a consultation session with a psychiatrist or another physician who can evaluate whether or not medication might be helpful. Some people worry about the effects of antidepressant medication. Some of the most common concerns are addressed here.

How Do I Know if Medication Will Help?

Approximately two of every three people who are depressed can be helped, to some degree, by antidepressant medication. There can be a trial-and-error process to prescribing antidepressants. Currently, there are dozens of antidepressants available, so you and your physician can't know with certainty which antidepressant will work for you until you've taken one for a few weeks. Different antidepressant medications may be prescribed depending on the particular symptoms you have and the specific effect you and your physician want to achieve. If the first antidepressant prescribed for you does not produce a beneficial effect, then your physician will try others until the desired effect is achieved. Unlike many other medications, antidepressants often take two to four weeks to achieve their beneficial effect. And because you may not respond positively to the initial medication prescribed for you, it may take eight weeks or longer to achieve therapeutic levels of the right antidepressants.

One drawback to antidepressants is annoying side effects, especially when one first begins to take antidepressants. The side effects include dry mouth, drowsiness, and weight changes, and they often diminish or disappear after the medication is taken for a period of time.

Does Taking Medication Mean I'm Crazy?

When we are depressed, the brain's supply of serotonin and/or norepinephrine, natural brain chemicals that affect thinking and moods, is decreased. Antidepressant medications help increase the levels of these chemicals, usually by blocking receptor sites, areas of the brain that break down these chemicals. The medications restore the brain to a more healthy, nondepressed state of serotonin or norepinephrine balance.

In fact, antidepressant medications work a lot like insulin for someone who is diabetic. Insulin is a natural chemical that diabetic people cannot produce in sufficient quantities for good health. Just as people who are diabetic take supplemental insulin to stay healthy, depressed people take supplemental medications to return to a natural state of good health. But unlike insulin for diabetics, most people do not have to take antidepressants forever.

Will I Become Addicted to the Medication?

Antidepressant medications are not addictive. However, it is important for you to follow your physician's directions in taking them because doses sometimes need to be increased and decreased and should be adjusted only according to medical guidelines.

Once you and your physician find an effective antidepressant, you will probably take it for six months to one year, although some people benefit from taking antidepressant medication longer, some even for several years. Your physician will help you evaluate how long you should take medication. In any case, when your physician recommends that you decrease antidepressant medication, you will not experience withdrawal symptoms as you would if these medications were addictive.

Improving Interpersonal Relationships

Some treatments for depression emphasize the importance of improving close relationships. If you are in an abusive relationship or a relationship with someone who criticizes you constantly, it can be hard to recover from depression. Couples therapy or family therapy can help you improve relationship conditions that may be feeding your depression. If you are being physically or sexually abused, almost all communities have special programs nearby to help you.

On the plus side, improving your relationships can help provide positive support as you recover from depression. The strategies taught in this book can be used to help you improve relationships that are already pretty good. Another self-help book that uses a cognitive therapy approach for couples' problems is Beck's *Love Is Never Enough* (New York: HarperCollins, 1988).

Activity Scheduling

Activities can be connected to the way you feel. If you track feelings of depression, you may discover that when you are depressed you are more passive and less active. Following the observation that depressed people tend to stop doing pleasurable activities, depression treatments often emphasize increasing the weekly number of pleasurable activities.

As a first step toward treating depression, it is often helpful to increase activities—especially pleasurable activities or those that lead to a sense of accomplishment. When we do activities that are enjoyable or activities that accomplish something, we usually feel better.

Depression reduces one's ability to concentrate, pay attention, and remember. If concentration, attention, and memory are affected so much that it is difficult to learn the cognitive interventions presented in this book, then it is best to focus exclusively on behavioral changes until concentration, attention, and memory have improved enough to learn the other skills.

By tracking your activities, you can discover how they affect your moods. You will see how your past and current activities are associated with your mood. And you will probably notice that your depression is reduced by planning future activities.

By scheduling and doing activities that are enjoyable or accomplish something, you will be making behavioral changes that can reduce your depression. Doing ten enjoyable activities in a week should help you more than doing only five. Additionally, doing activities that are highly enjoyable should help you more than doing activities that are mildly enjoyable. Different people enjoy different activities. Examples of enjoyable activities include talking to a friend, listening to music, playing a computer game, taking a walk, going out for lunch, watching a favorite TV show or sporting event, or playing with your child. Notice that pleasurable activities need not be expensive or time consuming. They are everyday enjoyable events.

If you decide to try activity scheduling as a first step in reducing your depression, do not expect to find the activities as enjoyable or as satisfying as you did before you became depressed. Ben, for example, who had greatly enjoyed golfing before he became depressed, found golfing a diversion during his depression but not as satisfying as it had been previously. If Ben had compared his golfing pleasure when depressed to his earlier enjoyment of this activity, he might have concluded, "This is no good. I'm not having fun like I used to." As a result of these thoughts, Ben might actually have felt more depressed after golfing. However, if Ben had compared his golfing enjoyment to sitting at home depressed, he might have decided, "It's good that I went golfing. At least I enjoyed myself a little bit. It was better than sitting at home feeling glum."

You can use a Weekly Activity Record to help you identify what you are doing when you feel most depressed, anxious, or angry. In addition to identifying your behavior and moods, the weekly activity schedule can be used as a guide to see what changes in your behavior might help you feel better.

EXERCISE: Activity Record

First, choose a mood that is troublesome for you or that occurs fairly recently and write this mood here:

Mood: _____

During this week, you will be rating this mood on a 0–100 point scale.

0	10	20	30	40	50	60	70	80	90	100

| Not at all | | A little | | | Medium | | | A lot | | Most I've ever felt |

Fill in your Weekly Activity Schedule (Worksheet 10.4 on pages 168–169) for one week. For each hour write in the activity you were doing and rate your mood on a scale from 0 to 100. You may forget to do it for some hours, but the more hours you fill in for the week, the more you will have a chance to learn about the mood you are rating. Therefore, if you forget to do it one day, don't give up—just continue the ratings when you remember.

Look at Ben's Weekly Activity Schedule in Figure 10.1 on pages 166–167. Notice that Ben wrote only a word or two to describe his activity—just enough to remind him what he was doing when he looked back at the record. When he did more than one activity in a time period, he wrote down the one or two most important behaviors (e.g., "walk," "breakfast,") or an overall word ("shopping").

Although Ben thought the Weekly Activity Schedule would be hard to keep, he found he needed just a few seconds each hour to put down an activity and a depression rating. Notice that on Thursday from 10:00 to 11:00 A.M., when his depression changed a lot during the hour, he wrote both a low and high rating to show the change.

To help you remember to fill out the Activity Schedule, carry a copy with you. It is not necessary to fill it out every hour. Most people can remember their moods for several hours, so you may be able to fill it out several times a day rather than hourly. For example, at lunch time you might write in all your morning activities and your mood ratings. At dinner time you might do the afternoon hours, at bedtime fill in the evening hours.

The connection between behavior and moods is important enough to suggest that you pause in reading this chapter until you have had a chance to fill out a Weekly Activity Schedule for a full week. Then continue reading this chapter. The remainder of the chapter will be more valuable to you if you can apply it to information you collected on your Weekly Activity Schedule.

REMINDER BOX

Weekly Activity Schedule

- Name the mood you will rate.

- Write down your activities for each hour of the day.

- For each hour, rate your mood.

- After filling out an activity schedule for one week, look for connections between what you do and your mood.

Write in each box: (1) Activity. (2) Mood ratings for depression (0–100%).

Time	MONDAY	TUESDAY	WEDNESDAY	THURSDAY	FRIDAY	SATURDAY	SUNDAY
6–7 A.M.	Wake up 60	Wake up 70	Wake up 60	Wake up 50	Wake up 60	Wake up 40	Wake up 60
7–8 A.M.	Shower, dress 60	Lie in bed 80	Shower, dress 50	Shower, dress 50	Dress 60	Shower, dress 30	Dress 60
8–9 A.M.	Walk, breakfast 40	Get dressed 80	Breakfast 50	Breakfast 40	Breakfast 40	Breakfast 20	Breakfast 50
9–10 A.M.	Golf 40	Breakfast 80	Hardware store 40	Walk 30	Clean garage 40	Drive to Bob's 20	Walk 40
10–11 A.M.	Golf 40	Sit in chair 80	Fix door 30	Phone call (Bob) 30–60	Clean garage 30	Visit with Bob and kids 10	Shopping 30
11–12 P.M.	Golf 60	Read 80	Fix door 30	Talk with Sylvie 60	Clean garage 30	Look at baseball cards with Greg 10	Shopping 30
12–1 P.M.	Lunch with Sylvie 40	Lunch with Sylvie 70	Lunch with Sylvie 20	Lunch 60	Lunch 20	Lunch 0	Lunch out 20
1–2 P.M.	Shopping with Sylvie 40	Wash dishes 80	Wash dishes 30	Therapy 50	Sweep garage 20	Go to park 0	Drive around with Sylvie 20
2–3 P.M.	Shopping 40	Sit in chair 80	Walk 20	Call Bert 40	Walk with Sylvie 20	Play catch 0	Home with Sylvie—relax 20

3–4 P.M.	Shopping 50	Pay bills 80	Read mail 20	Clean up workbench 40	Read newspaper, mail 20	Walk Bob's dog 0	Relax with Sylvie 10
4–5 P.M.	Unpack shopping bags 50	Drive Sylvie to bank 70	Help cook 20	Help cook 40	Help cook 20	Drive home 10	Make dinner 10
5–6 P.M.	Sit in chair 60	Dinner out 60	Dinner with Sylvie 20	Dinner 30	Dinner 20	Dinner 10	Dinner 10
6–7 P.M.	Dinner 60	Walk at shopping mall 60	Wash dishes 20	Wash dishes 30	Wash dishes 20	Wash dishes 10	Wash dishes 10
7–8 P.M.	TV 60	Movie 50	Play cards 20	TV 30	Phone call with Bob 10	Sat in chair 30	TV 20
8–9 P.M.	TV 60	Movie 50	Play cards 20	TV 40	TV 10	Look at photo album 30	TV 20
9–10 P.M.	TV 60	Drive home 50	Talk to Sylvie 20	TV 40	TV 10	Talk with Sylvie 20	TV 20
10–11 P.M.	TV 60	TV 50	TV 20	TV 40	TV 10	TV 30	TV 30
11–12 A.M.	Bed 70	Bed 60	Bed 20	Bed 60	Bed 10	Bed 30	Bed 20
12–1 A.M.	Sleep	Sleep	Sleep	Sleep	Sleep	Sleep	Sleep

FIGURE 10.1. Ben's Weekly Activity Schedule.

WORKSHEET 10.4: Tracking Activities—Weekly Activity Schedule

Write in each box: (1) Activity. (2) Mood ratings (0–100). (Mood I am rating: _____

Time	MONDAY	TUESDAY	WEDNESDAY	THURSDAY	FRIDAY	SATURDAY	SUNDAY
6–7 A.M.							
7–8 A.M.							
8–9 A.M.							
9–10 A.M.							
10–11 A.M.							
11–12 P.M.							
12–1 P.M.							
1–2 P.M.							
2–3 P.M.							

3–4 P.M.	4–5 P.M.	5–6 P.M.	6–7 P.M.	7–8 P.M.	8–9 P.M.	9–10 P.M.	10–11 P.M.	11–12 A.M.	12–1 A.M.

Complete the following exercise after you have filled out a Weekly Activity Schedule for one week.

Exercise: Learning from Activity Records

Now that you have charted your moods and activities for one week, analyze your Weekly Activity Schedule to look for patterns. Worksheet 10.5 lists some questions to answer to help you learn from your Weekly Activity Schedule.

WORKSHEET 10.5: Learning from the Weekly Activity Schedule

1. Did my mood change during the week? How? What patterns do I notice?

2. Did my activities affect my mood? How?

3. What activities helped me feel better? Why? Are these activities in my best long-term interest? What other activities could I do that might also make me feel better?

4. What activities helped me feel worse? Why? Are these activities in my best interest to do?

5. Were there certain times of the day (e.g., mornings) or week (e.g., weekends) when I felt worse?

6. Can I think of anything I could do to feel better during these times?

7. Were there certain times of the day or week when I felt better?

8. Looking at my answers to questions 3 and 4, what activities can I plan in the coming week to increase the chances that I will feel better this week? Over the next few months?

Your answers to Worksheet 10.5 can help you identify activities you might need to change in order to feel better. Refer to Ben's Weekly Activity Schedule (Figure 10.1) and see how he answered the questions on Worksheet 10.5 (Figure 10.2).

1. Did my mood change during the week? How? What patterns do I notice?

Yes, my mood changed. Once I get down, it seems to last for hours. Some days were not so bad.

2. Did my activities affect my mood? How?

Yes. On busy days I usually felt a little better.

3. What activities helped me feel better? Why? Are these activities in my best long-term interest? What other activities could I do that might also make me feel better?

Doing things with Sylvie—she is a happy person. Fixing the door—I felt useful. Yes. Spend time with grandchildren. Play more golf. Work in garden.

4. What activities helped me feel worse? Why? Are these activities in my best interest to do?

Sitting in my chair thinking—bad news.

Phone call from Bob on Thursday—bad news.

Yes, in my best interest—it is necessary to deal with difficult situations.

5. Were there certain times of the day (e.g., mornings) or week (e.g., weekends) when I felt worse?

Felt worse in the mornings until I got going.

Felt worse early in the week.

6. Can I think of anything I could do to feel better during these times?

I guess it helps when I shower, get dressed. Walking seems to help, although I don't feel like it when I'm down. Getting out of the house might help on bad days.

7. Were there certain times of the day or week I felt better?

Generally, later in the day I felt better. This week I felt better on Friday, Saturday, and Sunday.

8. Looking at my answers to questions 3 and 4, what activities can I plan in the coming week to increase the chances that I will feel better this week? Over the next few months?

Fix up things around the house. Plan more activities—especially fun things. Visit my grandchildren. Walk Bob's dog. Spend less time sitting alone.

FIGURE 10.2. What Ben learned from his Weekly Activity Schedule.

As you can see, Ben learned a lot from his Weekly Activity Schedule. Depending on the mood you tracked, you might have learned a variety of things from observing your own emotional shifts. Depressed people often observe that if they become more active, it helps them feel better. Why do you think this might be so?

_____

_____

_____

_____

We don't know for sure why depressed people often feel better after they start doing more things. Here is a list of possible reasons:

- Some types of activities, like exercise, increase the brain chemicals that can help us feel better.

- When we are doing nothing we are often thinking about negative things over and over again. Activity helps distract us from negative thoughts.

- Activities can give us the opportunity to succeed (e.g., organize a room or desk), to do something enjoyable (e.g., talk with someone we like), or to solve a problem (begin working on something that has to get done). Each of these experiences—success, joy, solving a problem—can help us feel a little better for awhile.

Activities seem to particularly help depression if they involve pleasure or a chance to accomplish something (even something very small). Therefore, just learning to look for pleasure or accomplishment in the things you do may help you feel better. In addition to looking at the effects of activity on your mood, try to see if any other changes in your behavior might help your mood. Ben and his therapist decided he should get up, get showered, and get dressed each morning, no matter how he felt—no lying in bed. Ben also decided to take a regular morning walk and to ask Sylvie to help him think of activities to do on the days he felt most depressed.

CHAPTER 10 SUMMARY

- Depression does not just describe a mood; it also involves changes in our thinking, behavior, and biology.

- The *Mind Over Mood* Depression Inventory (Worksheet 10.1) can be used to rate depression symptoms. Weekly scores on the inventory can be charted on Worksheet 10.2 to note changes in depression as you use this manual.

- Learning to change how you think is a main focus of cognitive therapy for depression.

- Medication can also be helpful, especially for people who experience intense or long-lasting depression.

- Rating your moods during activities, written down on a weekly activity schedule, can help you discover the connections between behavior and depression (Worksheet 10.4).

- Analyzing the Weekly Activity Schedule can suggest behavioral changes to make to help you feel better (Worksheet 10.5).

- Pleasurable activities or activities that allow you to accomplish something help you feel better when you are depressed.

CHAPTER 11

Understanding Anxiety

Anxiety is one of the most distressing emotions that people feel. It is sometimes called fear or nervousness. The word "anxiety" describes a number of problems including *phobias* (fear of specific things or situations, such as heights, elevators, insects, flying in airplanes), *panic attacks* (intense feelings of anxiety in which people often feel like they are about to die or go crazy), *posttraumatic stress disorder* (repeated, memories of terrible traumas with high levels of distress), *obsessive–compulsive disorder* (thinking about or doing things over and over again), and *generalized anxiety disorder* (a mixture of worries and anxiety symptoms experienced most of the time). We also use the word "anxiety" to describe brief periods of nervousness or fear we experience when faced with difficult experiences in our life.

Most people who are anxious are very aware of the physical symptoms, which can include jitteriness, tension, sweaty palms, light-headedness, difficulty breathing, increased heart rate, and flushed cheeks. Anxiety is similar to depression in that symptoms are experienced in the four areas described in Chapter 1.

ANXIETY PROFILE

Physical Reactions

Sweaty palms

Muscle tension

Racing heart

Flushed cheeks

Light-headedness

Thoughts

Overestimation of danger

Underestimation of your ability to cope

Underestimation of help available

Worries and catastrophic thoughts

Behaviors

Avoiding situations where anxiety might occur

Leaving situations when anxiety begins to occur

Trying to do things perfectly or trying to control events to prevent danger

Moods

Nervous

Irritable

Anxious

Panicky

Important events in our lives (environment) can contribute to anxiety. Examples of important events are trauma (e.g., being physically or sexually abused; being in an automobile accident; being in a war), illness or deaths, things we are taught ("Snakes will bite you," "If you get dirty, you'll get sick,"), things we observe (an article in the newspaper about a plane crash, "My heart just missed a beat"), and experiences that seem too much to handle (giving a public speech, job promotion or termination, having a new baby). Linda's anxiety began after her father's death. Linda felt overwhelmed and had greater difficulty coping with problems. She began to expect that another catastrophe would occur and that she would not be able to cope with it.

All the physical, behavioral, and thinking changes we experience when we are anxious are part of the anxiety responses called "fight, flight, or freeze." These three responses can be adaptive when we face danger. To see how this is so, imagine that you are out of town. You decide to go for a walk at night and find yourself lost on a dark street. You notice a large man approximately 20 yards away walking toward you. You believe that he sees you and think that he is going to attack and rob you. What should you do? One option would be to fight. To do this, your heart would pump faster, your breathing would speed up, and your muscles would tense. Sweating would help cool your body. As you can see, all these body changes would be helpful in this situation (but not so helpful when facing your boss—a social danger). These changes make up the "fight" response.

Maybe you do not think fighting the man is a good idea. Perhaps you think it would be better to run. To run fast, you would also need an accelerated heart rate, plenty of oxygen, muscle tension, and sweating. Therefore, the same physical changes that make up the "fight" response make up the "flight" response. You simply use the extra energy to run rather than to stay and do battle. With a little luck, running may save you from being attacked.

A third response that might work well would be to freeze. Maybe the man has not seen you, and perhaps if you are very still he will not notice you. In this case, a total freeze would require you to have very tense, rigid muscles. With a tight chest you would not even breath very visibly. The types of physical changes that cause you to be very still are part of the "freeze" response.

These three anxiety responses—fight, flight, and freeze—are good reactions to danger. Unfortunately, we also experience these reactions when watching a movie about a robbery or when standing in front of a group of people to give a speech. This book teaches methods to reduce your anxiety when danger is not present, when the danger is not as serious as you might think, or when too much anxiety interferes with good coping.

As described in Chapter 1, Linda had anxiety and panic attacks on her way to the airport, while in the boarding area, and on entering an airplane. Her heartbeat was rapid, she sweated, her breathing changed and her muscles tensed, symptoms that led her to believe that she was in danger of having a heart attack.

To get a better picture of your own anxiety, write down the types of events or situations in which you tend to feel anxious:

I feel anxious when _____

I also feel anxious when _____

I also feel anxious when _____

I also feel anxious when _____

EXERCISE: Identifying and Assessing Symptoms of Anxiety

To specify what symptoms you experience when you are anxious, rate the symptoms listed in the *Mind Over Mood* Anxiety Inventory on Worksheet 11.1 on page 178. Fill out the inventory once or twice per week while you are learning methods to manage your anxiety in order to determine which interventions are most effective.

Score the *Mind Over Mood* Anxiety Inventory by adding up the numbers you circled for all the items. For example, if you circled 3 for each item your score would be 72 (3 X 24 items). If you couldn't decide between two numbers for an item and circled both, add only the higher number.

To chart change, record your *Mind Over Mood* Anxiety Inventory scores on Worksheet 11.2 on page 179. Mark each column with the date you made out the *Mind Over Mood* Anxiety Inventory. Then put an X in the column across from your score.

COGNITIVE ASPECTS OF ANXIETY

The thoughts that accompany anxiety are different from the thoughts that characterize depression. Anxiety is accompanied by the perception that we are in DANGER or that we are THREATENED or VULNERABLE in some way. As you learned earlier in this chapter, the physical symptoms of anxiety prepare us to respond to the danger or threat we expect.

A threat or danger can be physical, mental, or social. A physical threat occurs when you believe you will be physically hurt (e.g., a snake bite, a heart attack, being hit). A social threat occurs when you believe you will be rejected, humiliated, embarrassed, or put down. A mental threat occurs when something makes you worry that you are going crazy or losing your mind.

The perception of threat varies from person to person. Some people, because of their life experiences, may feel threatened very easily and will often feel anxious. Other people may feel a greater sense of safety and security. Growing up in chaotic and volatile surroundings may lead a person to conclude that the world and other people are continually and constantly dangerous.

The perception of danger and a sense of your own vulnerability may have helped you survive as a child. If you grew up in a dangerous home, being able to recognize danger or its early warning signs were critical to your emotional and perhaps your physical survival. You may have developed a very fine ability to spot and respond to dangerous situations.

WORKSHEET 11.1 *Mind Over Mood* Anxiety Inventory

Circle one number for each item that best describes how much you have experienced each symptom over the past week.

	Not at all	Sometimes	Frequently	Most of the time
1. Feeling nervous	0	1	2	3
2. Frequent worrying	0	1	2	3
3. Trembling, twitching, feeling shaky	0	1	2	3
4. Muscle tension, muscle aches, muscle soreness	0	1	2	3
5. Restlessness	0	1	2	3
6. Easily tired	0	1	2	3
7. Shortness of breath	0	1	2	3
8. Rapid heartbeat	0	1	2	3
9. Sweating not due to the heat	0	1	2	3
10. Dry mouth	0	1	2	3
11. Dizziness or light-headedness	0	1	2	3
12. Nausea, diarrhea, or stomach problems	0	1	2	3
13. Frequent urination	0	1	2	3
14. Flushes (hot flashes) or chills	0	1	2	3
15. Trouble swallowing or "lump in throat"	0	1	2	3
16. Feeling keyed up or on edge	0	1	2	3
17. Quick to startle	0	1	2	3
18. Difficulty concentrating	0	1	2	3
19. Trouble falling or staying asleep	0	1	2	3
20. Irritability	0	1	2	3
21. Avoiding places where I might be anxious	0	1	2	3
22. Frequent thoughts of danger	0	1	2	3
23. Seeing myself as unable to cope	0	1	2	3
24. Frequent thoughts that something terrible will happen	0	1	2	3

Score (of total circled numbers) ☐

WORKSHEET 11.2: *Mind Over Mood Anxiety Inventory Scores*

Score																					
72																					
69																					
66																					
63																					
60																					
57																					
54																					
51																					
48																					
45																					
42																					
39																					
36																					
33																					
30																					
27																					
24																					
21																					
18																					
15																					
12																					
9																					
6																					
3																					
0																					
Date																					

At this point in your life, it may be important to evaluate whether or not you are overresponding to danger and threat. Perhaps the people in your adult life are not as threatening as those in your childhood. You might also consider whether or not your resources and abilities as an adult open new and creative ways of responding to threat and anxiety.

Anxious thoughts are future oriented and often predict catastrophe. Anxious thoughts often begin with "What if . . . " and end with a disastrous outcome. Anxious thoughts frequently include images of danger, as well. For example, a man with a fear of public speaking may, before a talk, think, "*What if* I stumble over my words? *What if* I forget my notes? *What if* people think I'm a fool and don't know what I'm talking about?" He may have an image of himself standing frozen in front of the crowd. These thoughts are all about the future and they all predict a dire outcome.

Someone who is afraid of flying in airplanes or driving on the freeway may think, "*What if* the airplane explodes? *What if* I have a panic attack on the airplane? *What if* there's not enough oxygen on the plane to breathe? *What if* I have a traffic accident on the freeway?, *What if* I get stuck in rush-hour traffic, have difficulty breathing and can't get to a freeway exit?" You can see that these thoughts are future oriented and predict danger or catastrophe: they would make you think twice about getting on an airplane or freeway.

Some people feel anxious in close relationships. They may fear intimacy or commitment. They may also be concerned about being judged, rejected, or embarrassed. The thoughts we have when we are fearful about relationships are also oriented to the future and predict danger or catastrophe. These thoughts might include "*What if* I get hurt?, *What if* I am rejected?, *What if* the other person senses my weakness and takes advantage of me?" These thoughts demonstrate the "something terrible is going to happen" theme that is characteristic of anxiety.

EXERCISE: Identifying Thoughts Associated with Anxiety

To highlight the thoughts that are associated with anxiety or fear in your own life, complete Worksheet 11.3 (recognize it? It's the first three columns of a Thought Record as described in Chapter 4). Think about a recent time when you were anxious, fearful, or nervous. Recall the thoughts you had (in words, in images). If you had a visual image, describe it. If your thoughts were in words, notice if the thoughts began with "What if...".

Were these thoughts you identified in the exercise future oriented? Do the thoughts imply some danger, vulnerability, or predict a catastrophe? If so, then you have identified anxiety-related thoughts.

WORKSHEET 11.3.   Identifying Thoughts Associated with Anxiety

1. Situation	2. Moods	3. Automatic Thoughts (Images)
Who? What? When? Where?	**a.** What did you feel? **b.** Rate each mood (0–100%).	**a.** What was going though your mind just before you started to feel this way? Any other thoughts? Images? **b.** Circle the hot thought.

COGNITIVE ASPECTS OF PANIC

Panic is extreme anxiety or fear. A panic attack consists of a distinct combination of emotions and physical symptoms. Often a panic attack is characterized by a change in bodily or mental sensations, such as rapid heartbeat, sweating, difficulty breathing, a choking or smothering sensation, shaking, dizziness, pain in the chest, nausea, hot flashes or chills, or disorientation.

While many people experience a panic attack at least once in their lifetime, some people develop panic disorder. They experience frequent panic attacks in which they are convinced each time that they are about to die. The key thoughts in panic disorder are catastrophic misinterpretations of body or mental sensations. For example, a rapid heartbeat may be misinterpreted as a heart attack. Being momentarily disoriented may be misinterpreted as going crazy. It is not uncommon for people with panic disorder to go to a hospital emergency room, only to discover that they are healthy and in no danger.

In people with panic disorder, a vicious circle occurs in which physical symptoms, emotions, and thoughts interact with each other and escalate rapidly. For example, if a woman susceptible to panic attacks notices that her heart is beating more rapidly than "normal," she may think, "Maybe I'm having a heart attack." This thought leads to fear and anxiety and stimulates the release of adrenaline. The release of adrenaline further accelerates her heart rate, which can convince her that she is experiencing a heart attack. Thoughts about physical sensations can actually make the sensations more intense. Catastrophic thoughts and the more intense physical and emotional reactions which follow can lead to avoidance of activities or situations in which previous panic attacks occurred.

Linda had to fly to a city 200 miles away for an impromptu business meeting. She monitored her thoughts and emotional reactions before the flight and summarized them in the Thought Record shown in Figure 11.1.

Notice how Linda's anxiety and panic were influenced by thoughts that focused on danger and personal vulnerability. It was not waiting in the airline terminal that caused Linda to panic. Many people wait in airline terminals without feeling anxious or having panic attacks. Linda's thoughts of the situation brought on her emotional reaction.

1. Situation	2. Moods	3. Automatic Thoughts (Images)
Who? What? When? Where?	**a.** What did you feel? **b.** Rate each mood (0–100%)	**a.** What was going though your mind just before you started to feel this way? Any other thoughts? Images? **b.** Circle the hot thought
Waiting in the airport to board my plane	*Anxiety 80%* *Panic 90%*	*What if the plane has engine trouble? How safe can this plane be? What if I have a panic attack on the plane?* *I'll be so embarrassed if my boss sees that I'm having trouble breathing and that I'm sweating and panicking. My heart is starting to race already.* *I think the panic attack is beginning.* *What if I have a heart attack?* *Image—I see myself grabbing my chest, sweating, and turning pale. People on the airplane are yelling.*

From *Mind Over Mood* by Dennis Greenberger and Christine A. Padesky. © 1995 The Guilford Press.

FIGURE 11.1. Linda's Thought Record.

OVERCOMING ANXIETY

The cognitive methods described in this book are highly effective in reducing and managing anxiety. Most people are able to stop their panic attacks by identifying and altering the thoughts that accompany panic.In addition to cognitive interventions, many people find relaxation training, imagery and behavioral methods helpful in alleviating anxiety. This section briefly describes each of these methods.

Cognitive Restructuring

Anxiety can be reduced either by decreasing your perception of danger or increasing your confidence in the ability to cope with threat. Chapters 4 to 7 teach you how to evaluate your anxious thoughts so that you can more quickly evaluate the danger and its consequences. Anxiety may decrease if you examine the evidence and discover that the danger you face is not as bad as you thought. When threats or dangers are present, it is helpful to figure out what strategies will best help cope with them (Chapter 8). Therefore, cognitive restructuring for anxiety involves both evaluating your estimations of danger and improving your awareness of coping options.

For panic disorder, cognitive restructuring is the central feature of successful therapy. If you suffer from panic attacks, your therapist will help you identify your catastrophic fears concerning specific body or mental sensations. Once you have identified these fears, you will do experiments (Chapter 8) to help you learn and believe in alternative noncatastrophic explanations for these sensations.

Relaxation Training

Relaxation training can be divided into methods that focus on physical relaxation and methods that focus on mental relaxation. All methods can be equally effective. Experiment with several and use the process that works best for you. When we are physically relaxed, mental relaxation follows, and when we are mentally relaxed, physical relaxation follows. Relaxation training can alleviate anxiety because it is difficult for the body or mind to be simultaneously relaxed and anxious. If you develop the ability to relax before and during stressful situations, then you can substantially reduce the frequency and severity of the anxiety you experience.

Progressive Muscle Relaxation

Progressive muscle relaxation is a technique in which the major muscle groups in the body are alternately tensed and relaxed. The process can proceed from the head to the feet or from the feet to the head. Progressive muscle relaxation can lead to deep levels of physical and mental relaxation. One tenses and relaxes the muscles in the forehead, eyes, jaws, neck, shoulders, upper back, biceps, forearms, hands, abdomen, groin, legs, hips, thighs, buttocks, calves and feet. Each muscle group is tensed for 5 seconds and then relaxed for 10 to 15 seconds, tensed for 5 seconds, relaxed for 10 to 15 seconds.

Different people carry muscle tension in different parts of their bodies, so the particular areas that need emphasis vary from person to person. Most people report increased levels of relaxation and decreased levels of physical tension and anxiety on completing a progressive muscle relaxation exercise. Repeated practice of any relaxation method creates even deeper levels of relaxation. Relaxation is a skill that can be developed much like playing the piano or throwing a ball. The more one practices, the greater the development of the skill.

Controlled Breathing

A second type of relaxation training is called controlled breathing. This method is based on the observation that many people breathe shallowly or irregularly when anxious or tense. These breathing patterns lead to an imbalance of oxygen and carbon dioxide in the body, which can cause the physical symptoms of anxiety.

It is important to practice controlled breathing for at least 4 minutes, because this is roughly how long it takes to restore the balance of oxygen and carbon dioxide. The balancing works most effectively if you breathe deeply in and out an equal amount of time. If you put one hand on your upper chest and one hand on your stomach, the hand on your stomach moves out as you breathe in.

Try breathing in to a slow count of 4 and out to a slow count of 4 for 4 minutes right now and see if you become more relaxed. It doesn't matter whether you breathe through your mouth or your nose; breathe whichever way is comfortable for you. Be sure to breathe gently and not take big gulps of air.

Imagery

Imagery methods are also effective for learning to relax and manage anxiety. Imagery involves actively visualizing scenes that are tranquil and relaxing to you. Scenes may be actual places you know that feel safe and relaxing, or they may be scenes you create to be tranquil, safe, and relaxing. The specific scene is less important than how the image makes you feel.

The more senses you can incorporate into your image, the more relaxing imagery is likely to be. If you can imagine the smells, sounds, and tactile sensations as well as the visual aspects of the scene, you will improve your ability to relax. For example, if you imagine yourself walking along a tree-lined mountain path, you may want to focus your attention on the birds singing, the light dancing through the tree branches, the smell of pine, the greenness of the forest, and the cool breeze as it touches your skin. Each one of our senses can contribute to our experience of relaxation and comfort.

Distraction

A fourth method of reducing the frequency and severity of anxiety is distraction. When anxious, we tend to focus on physical sensations or thoughts connected to our anxiety. Distraction works because our attention is focused away from the thoughts or physical sensations that contribute to our anxiety.

To the degree that you can become absorbed in other activities or thoughts you will shut off the cognitive fuel for your anxiety, thereby decreasing or eliminating your anxiety symptoms. The more fully you are able to absorb yourself in other thoughts or activities, the more your anxiety will dissipate. Like controlled breathing, it is important to practice distraction for at least 4 minutes before expecting a decrease in anxiety.

Linda learned to use distraction effectively in the early phases of her therapy. Linda was on an airplane when the pilot announced that the plane would be delayed on the runway for 20 minutes. Linda's initial thoughts were "I won't be able to handle this. I'll have a panic attack," and she began to experience anxiety. Although she had learned progressive muscle relaxation and how to use Thought Records, Linda decided to experiment with distraction.

Linda began to focus her attention on the sky and clouds. She concentrated on the shades of blue in the sky and on the colors and shapes of the clouds. She allowed her eyes to run over the outlines of the clouds and to observe closely the texture of each cloud. Additionally, she sought to amuse herself by looking for pictures in the clouds; she was surprised to find that many of them resembled cartoon characters. Linda became so absorbed in the scene that the 20-minute delay went by quickly with virtually no anxiety.

You may want to try each of these relaxation methods once or twice to see which ones work best for you. To determine which relaxation methods work best for you, rate your level of anxiety or tension on a 0–100 scale before and after completing them. Many people find that distraction is the best method for very high levels of anxiety and that the other methods work well at medium levels of anxiety. Practice the one or two methods that work best for you regularly to make them fully effective.

Overcoming Avoidance

Avoidance is a hallmark of anxiety. When we avoid a difficult situation, we initially experience a decrease in anxiety. Ironically, the more we avoid a situation, the more anxious we become about facing it in the future. In this way, avoidance in the long run actually feeds anxiety, even though it seems to help anxiety in the short run. To overcome anxiety, we need to learn to approach the situations or people we avoid. Learning to approach and cope with situations in which we feel anxious is a lasting and powerful way of eliminating anxiety.

In order to approach feared situations successfully, you can use the relaxation skills described in this chapter to reduce your anxiety about the situations. By gradually approaching what you fear, you can gather evidence about the accuracy of your catastrophic expectations.

If you experience high levels of anxiety, it is helpful to develop a hierarchy of the situations, events, or people you fear. A hierarchy is a list written in order of fear intensity, with the most feared situation or event at the top and the least feared event at the bottom. Start to approach situations on the bottom of the list first and work up the list gradually, successfully mastering and approaching events that are not as frightening before approaching the most feared situation.

As an example, Juanita was nervous because she had been asked to give a presentation at the next city council meeting. She usually avoided speaking in front of groups because she felt so anxious. To overcome her anxiety and avoidance, Juanita made a hierarchy that looked like this:

5. Speaking at the city council meeting.

4. Meeting privately with one council member to present my ideas.

3. Giving my speech to family and friends.

2. Practicing the presentation at home alone.

1. Writing the speech.

Starting with situation 1, Juanita successfully met the challenges of each situation in the hierarchy by combining relaxation methods, cognitive restructuring (Chapters 4–7), and Action Plans (Chapter 8) to solve problems that might occur. Juanita did not proceed to the next situation in her hierarchy until she could approach the previous one with little or no anxiety. She practiced step 4—a step that could not be easily repeated numerous times—in her imagination until she experienced minimal anxiety. While Juanita experienced some anxiety when she actually gave her presentation to the City

Council, she was not nearly as anxious as she had been in similar situations in the past. She credited her success to her step-by-step practice. Further, as Juanita walked to the podium, she reminded herself how well she had done the speech in practice. By using different methods in combination, Juanita was able to give a public speech, an event she had previously avoided.

When you use a hierarchy, you have control over how quickly or slowly you proceed through your list of events. Your exposure to the events is self-initiated, and you should not feel pushed or pressured to go faster than you believe you can. Having a sense of control over the speed at which you work is critical in your ultimate mastery of the events.

If you find that even the least feared situation on the hierarchy seems too difficult, you can either break down that event into smaller pieces or begin with imagery practice. Imagery practice is simply picturing oneself completing the step. While you imagine the situation, you can use cognitive restructuring and relaxation methods to reduce the level of anxiety that is stimulated by your imagery. Once you are comfortable with the situation in imagination, you can enter the situation in reality.

Sometimes a supportive spouse, friend, or partner can help you be more willing and motivated to face your fear hierarchy. If you want a partner to help, choose someone you trust and who understands the nature of your fears and avoidance. This person can serve as an empathic source of motivation and support as you do initially difficult activities. Ideally, you will progress to face your fears on your own as well as with a friend.

Medication

Whereas medication is often indicated in the treatment of depression, its use in treating anxiety is more controversial. The medications most often recommended in treating anxiety are tranquilizers. Currently, the three most popular tranquilizers are Xanax™ (alprazolam), Valium™ (diazepam), and Klonopin™ (clonazepam). Most people agree that these medications can be helpful for short-term—up to 2 weeks—alleviation of anxiety symptoms. However, tranquilizers, unlike antidepressants, have a serious addiction potential. Further, tranquilizers can interfere with developing coping skills to overcome avoidance and manage anxiety without medication.

Tranquilizers produce pleasant, relaxed, calm sensations. People who take tranquilizers for an extended period of time may develop a tolerance, which means that it takes greater and greater amounts of the tranquilizer to produce a relaxed effect. Additionally, after taking tranquilizers for an extended period of time, many people experience withdrawal symptoms if they suddenly stop taking medication. Withdrawal symptoms include nausea, sweating, jitteriness, and an intense craving for the medication. Withdrawal and tolerance are two of the primary characteristics of addiction. This is why your physician will monitor you closely if you are on these medications. This is also why your physician may have recommended this book to help you learn other methods to reduce your anxiety.

Tranquilizers produce a rapid alleviation of anxiety, but they diminish the opportunity to learn, practice, and develop new skills. To develop methods to manage anxiety, you need to feel anxious and learn how to reduce the emotion. You cannot fully gauge the effects of deep breathing, cognitive restructuring, distraction, progressive muscle relaxation, and overcoming avoidance if you are taking tranquilizers. The motivation to learn new coping strategies is enhanced by high levels of anxiety. When one is very anxious, the desire to learn new methods to manage anxiety is very high. Since tranquilizers produce pleasant, pleasurable sensations, motivation to learn something new diminishes.

The effectiveness of any intervention, including medication, is measured by relapse rates as well as by immediate effect. Relapse rates record the number of people initially helped by an intervention who reexperience the same symptoms when the treatment is discontinued. Unfortunately, people with anxiety disorders, treated only with medication, experience high rates of relapse. For example, one study found that 71–95% of people with panic disorder whose panic was successfully treated with medication reexperienced panic attacks within 90 days after discontinuing the medication (Sheehan, 1986).* Other studies consistently find high relapse rates in patients whose panic disorder is treated only with medication. In contrast, studies of patients treated with cognitive therapy for panic disorder show cognitive therapy is an equally effective treatment with a relapse rate of only 0–10% up to one year after the end of treatment. Cognitive therapy teaches skills for conquering panic that lead to more permanent improvement.

The problems associated with tranquilizer use have led to the use of other types of medication. BuSpar® (Buspirone), one of the newest antianxiety medications, is nonsedating and, to date, seems nonaddictive; there are no withdrawal symptoms with discontinuance. Unlike tranquilizers, BuSpar is not effective if taken on an occasional basis. It is only effective when taken on a regular basis for at least a week.

It is interesting to note that antidepressant medications are sometimes used to treat anxiety. Antidepressants do not always help anxiety but, when they do, they have the advantage of being nonaddictive and the disadvantage of taking several weeks to reach therapeutic doses (see Chapter 10).

*Sheehan, D. V. (1986). Tricyclic antidepressants in the treatment of panic and anxiety disorders. *Psychosomatica*, *27*, 10–16.

The exception to these general anxiety medication guidelines is in the treatment of obsessive-compulsive disorder (OCD). OCD is characterized by persistent thoughts, impulses, or ideas that are disturbing and occur repeatedly. Often, the thoughts are followed by compulsive behaviors performed in response to the thoughts. For example, people with OCD may wash their hands 50 times in a row to reduce anxiety about disease, or they may drive around a block 25 times to be sure they did not hit a pedestrian. No matter how many times they do these behaviors, the anxiety is only temporarily reduced, if at all.

Research suggests that the best treatment for OCD may be a combination of medication (e.g., Anafranil™ or Prozac™) with behavioral therapy. For a description of the behavioral treatment of OCD, refer to *When Once Is Not Enough* by Gail Steketee and Kerrin White (Oakland, CA: New Harbinger Press, 1990). Although medication has proved more helpful in the long-term treatment of OCD than in the long-term treatment of any other anxiety problem, it is not a complete solution even for this type of anxiety. Medication typically will reduce OCD symptoms by half; psychological treatment (usually using behavioral or cognitive methods) is necessary to successfully treat the complete OCD problem.

CHAPTER 11 SUMMARY

- Anxiety disorders include phobias, panic attacks, posttraumatic stress disorder, obsessions, compulsions, and generalized anxiety.

- Anxiety symptoms include muscle tension, rapid heartbeat, light-headedness, avoidance, and nervousness.

- Cognitive components of anxiety include the perception of danger, vulnerability, or threat.

- Thoughts that accompany anxiety often begin with "What if . . . " and contain the theme that "something terrible is going to happen."

- Panic is extreme anxiety accompanied by catastrophic misinterpretations of body or mental sensations such as "I'm having a heart attack," "I'm dying," or "I'm losing my mind."

- Anxiety can be diminished or eliminated by cognitive restructuring, relaxation training, and overcoming avoidance.

CHAPTER 12

Understanding Anger, Guilt, and Shame

Anger, guilt, and shame are problematic for many people. Vic's difficulties in controlling his anger created significant problems in his marriage. Marissa's shame centered on her history of sexual abuse and affected her self-esteem and her relationships. This chapter describes the cognitive components of anger, guilt, and shame and details strategies for understanding and managing these feelings.

ANGER

Chapter 6 began with a description of Vic's angry explosion following a conversation with his wife, Judy. You may or may not express anger as Vic did, but you probably have experienced a similar upheaval of anger at times when you thought you were being seriously mistreated or someone was taking advantage of you. When we are angry, our body mobilizes for defense or attack, and our thoughts are often filled with plans for retaliation, or "getting even," or they focus on how "unfairly" we have been treated. As with all moods, anger is accompanied by changes in thinking, behavior, and physical functioning, as described in Chapter 1.

ANGER PROFILE

Thoughts

Others are threatening or hurtful

Rules have been violated

Others are treating me unfairly

Physical Reactions

Tight muscles

Increased blood pressure

Increased heart rate

Behaviors

Defend/Resist

Attack/Argue

Withdraw (to punish or protect)

Moods

Irritable

Angry

Enraged

Notice that the emotion of anger can range from irritation to rage. How angry we become in a given situation (social environment) is influenced by our interpretation of the meaning of the event. If Vic's wife, Judy, grew silent in a conversation and he interpreted her reaction as fatigue, Vic might be mildly irritated. However, if Vic thought Judy's silence meant that she didn't care for him or was belittling his concerns, Vic would feel much angrier.

There is great individual variation in the type of event that elicits anger. One person may get angry standing in line and yet listen calmly to criticisms of job performance. A different person may be perfectly content to stand in line and yet quickly attack anyone who points out work flaws. The types of events that provoke our anger are usually linked to our past as well as to rules and beliefs that we hold.

For example, if we have been abused frequently or severely in the past, we may have a tendency to be "on guard" against future abuse. We have learned that it is adaptive to be alert and wary of abuse if others are frequently hurting us. Some people who have a long history of abuse are quick to see current events as abusive and may experience chronic anger, sometimes seemingly out of proportion to the events that provoke the anger.

The pattern of quick and frequent anger goes along with a belief that it is possible to protect ourselves by confronting abuse. What about people who have been frequently abused but who feel helpless to protect themselves? People who believe they are helpless often react to abuse not with anger but with resignation or depression. For these people, the challenge may be to learn to experience anger when someone is directly harming them, rather than learning to control anger. Anger can be a problem, therefore, either because it is too frequent or because it is absent. It is normal to feel angry sometimes.

Exercise: Understanding Anger

To understand what happens when you are angry, remember a recent time when you felt angry or irritated. Describe the situation in column 1 of the Thought Record in Worksheet 12.1. On a 0–100 scale, with 100 being enraged, 50 being angry, and 10 being mildly irritated, rate your anger and describe it in a word or two in column 2.

At the point when you were most angry, what was going through your mind?

Write these thoughts (words, images, memories) in column 3.

If your anger reactions are troublesome to you, repeat this exercise for several other recent situations in which you have been angry. Describe the situations, rate the intensity of your anger, and then write down your thoughts, including any images you may have had. Once you have done this exercise for several situations, proceed to the next two sections, which describe a cognitive understanding of anger and outline approaches to help you harness your anger so that it can serve you constructively rather than destructively.

Cognitive Aspects of Anger

Anger is linked to a perception of damage or hurt and to a belief that important rules have been violated. We become angry if we think we have been treated unfairly, hurt unnecessarily, or prevented from obtaining something we expected to achieve. Notice the emphasis on fairness, reasonableness, and expectation. It is not simply the hurt or damage that makes us angry, but the violation of rules and expectations.

Imagine a man who loses his job. Does he feel angry? It depends. If the man loses his job and considers this a fair decision (perhaps because he broke company rules or the company went bankrupt), he is unlikely to feel angry.

However, if the man thinks his job loss was unfair (perhaps others broke rules and were not fired or only men of a certain race lost their jobs), then he probably feels very angry.

Similarly, if a child steps on your foot while you are riding on a bus, you feel pain. Whether or not you feel angry depends on your interpretation of

■ **WORKSHEET 12.1: Understanding Anger**

1. Situation	2. Moods	3. Automatic Thoughts (Images)
Who? What? When? Where?	a. What did you feel? b. Rate each mood (0–100%).	a. What was going though your mind just before you started to feel this way? Any other thoughts? Images? b. Circle the hot thought.

the intent and reasonableness of the child's behavior. Your anger is likely to be quick if you think the injury was intentional. But if you think that the child stepped on your foot by accident when a swerve of the bus made the child lose balance, you wince in pain but probably do not feel anger. The probability of anger in response to an unintentional injury is related to your judgments of "reasonableness." For example, on an overcrowded bus, we overlook someone stepping on our foot more easily than we do on a nearly empty bus.

These rules of anger seem quite straightforward until you consider that people vary greatly in what they consider fair and reasonable expectations. Vic expected Judy to be attentive and supportive to him even when he was behaving in ways she considered hurtful. Judy expected Vic to speak calmly to her even when he was feeling enraged. Both Vic and Judy believed that their own expectations were reasonable and the other's expectations were too perfectionistic.

As Vic and Judy discovered, anger is most likely to emerge in close relationships. Whether with a love partner or a work colleague, anger is rarely so intense as when it is experienced with someone with whom we are in close contact. The link between anger and intimacy can be best understood by recognizing that each of us has multiple expectations for our friendships, love relationships, work partnerships, and so forth. We are less likely to have specific personal expectations for people we meet casually. The closer our relationship with someone, the more likely we are to have expectations of them. To complicate the picture, we rarely tell people about our expectations, or even become aware of them ourselves, until they have been broken. Then we feel hurt, disappointed, and often angry.

Anger Management Strategies

Cognitive Restructuring

The cognitive restructuring methods taught in *Mind Over Mood* (Chapters 4–7) often help reduce anger. Other methods that may help you control your anger include anticipating and preparing for events that place you at high risk for experiencing anger, recognizing the early warning signs of anger, timeouts, assertion training and couples therapy.

Anticipating and Preparing for Events Using Imagery

You may find it helpful to anticipate situations in which you are likely to get angry and to prepare for them. The imagery methods to alleviate anxiety described in Chapter 11 can be helpful in minimizing the possibility of destructive anger. It is best to use imagery before entering a situation. You may find it helpful to imagine yourself saying what you want to say, in the manner in which you want to say it, and getting the response you hope to get. Further, it may be helpful to imagine how you can handle problems that might occur in an effective and adaptive way. Imagery works, in part, because it helps you think through possible problem areas and design your response in advance. Further, it can be helpful to see yourself as effective and relaxed in a high-risk, stressful situation. Finally, it is helpful to construct an ideal image of how you want to respond; the image can help guide your responses in the actual situation.

If you can identify a situation that is going to be stressful and in which you are at high risk for experiencing anger, you have the opportunity to plan, write out, and rehearse exactly what you want to say and how you want to say it. This script can help you develop a strategy targeted to what you want to achieve and enter the situation with a greater degree of confidence.

Recognizing Early Warning Signs of Anger

In addition to the anticipation of situations in which you are likely to be angry, it is also helpful to recognize the signs that you are becoming angry or that your anger is getting out of control. By recognizing these signs, you have the opportunity to short-circuit any destructive anger. Since anger can be helpful or destructive, if you learn to recognize when you are beginning to move into the destructive zone, you can then utilize various methods to reassert control and make your anger work constructively.

For many people, early warning signs of destructive anger include shakiness, muscle tension, clenched jaw, chest pressure, yelling, clenched fists, and saying things that are not true. When you become aware of any of these signals, it is important to take a moment to remind yourself of your options. You can choose to be angry or to use some of the methods described here to calm down.

Timeouts

Timeouts can be an effective way to control your anger. Taking a timeout involves removing yourself from the situation you are in when the early warning signs indicate that your anger is going out of control. Taking a timeout helps you reclaim control over yourself and over the situation.

The effective use of timeouts involves recognizing the earliest signs that your anger is getting out of control or is becoming destructive. You can use timeouts as athletes do to regroup, strategize, relax, or simply rest. Your timeout may be as short as 5 minutes or as long as 24 hours. The timeout is not used to avoid a situation but, rather, to approach the situation from a new angle and with a fresh start. The point of every timeout is to return to the situation and see it through.

You may want to enhance the timeout by using cognitive restructuring methods taught in this book (Chapters 4–7). At times, merely getting out of the situation helps to view it differently. You may also find it helpful to practice the relaxation exercises described in Chapter 11. Some people try to re-enter the situation with a new strategy to minimize the possibility of an angry blowup.

Assertion Training

Assertion training can reduce difficulties with anger. Assertion can reduce the frequency of being treated unfairly or being taken advantage of and, therefore, can prevent situations that give rise to anger.

Further, assertion training is helpful for people who hold anger in, internalizing the destructive effects of anger. For more information on learning to be assertive, not just angry, read *Your Perfect Right* by Robert Alberti and Michael Emmons (6th ed., 1990. San Luis Obispo, CA: Impact).

Couples Therapy

If anger management strategies do not effectively help you handle anger in your love relationships, couples therapy can help. Perceptions, attitudes, beliefs, and thoughts about your partner can fuel your anger. Therapy can teach couples how to communicate better, to increase positive interactions in the relationship, and to develop negotiation skills and strategies for identifying and altering expectations and rules. These skills can reduce relationship anger and improve the quality of your relationship with your partner. *Love Is Never Enough* by Aaron T. Beck (New York: Harper Collins, 1988) describes and outlines solutions to the difficulties couples frequently encounter.

GUILT AND SHAME

Guilt and shame are closely connected emotions. We tend to feel guilty when we have violated rules that are important to us or when we have not lived up to standards that we have set for ourselves. We feel guilty when we judge

ourselves to have done something wrong. If we think we "should" have behaved differently or that we "ought" to have done better, we are likely to feel
guilt.

Shame involves the sense that we have done something wrong. However, when we feel ashamed we assume that what we have done wrong
means that we are "flawed," "no good," "inadequate," "rotten," "awful,"
or "bad." Shame is usually connected to a highly negative view of ourselves. Secretiveness often surrounds shame. We may think, "If others knew
this secret they would hate me or think less of me." For this reason the
source of shame is rarely revealed and remains hidden and destructive.
Shame often accompanies a family secret involving other family members,
a secret such as alcoholism, sexual abuse, abortion, bankruptcy, or behavior considered dishonorable in the community.

Marissa's shame, for example, centered on her history of being sexually abused. Although the abuse began when she was 6 years old, Marissa
never fully revealed the extent of her abuse until she was 26 years old. She
attempted to tell her mother about the abuse when she was younger but
was scolded and accused of lying. Whenever Marissa had memories of the
sexual abuse she was overwhelmed by feelings of shame. While in therapy,
Marissa started a Thought Record that demonstrated the connection between her thoughts and her shame (Figure 12.1 on page 199). This example
demonstrates the secretive nature of shame ("I could never tell Julie this
happened") as well as how shame is connected to Marissa's view of herself as "awful" and "despicable."

Overcoming Guilt and Shame

Overcoming guilt and shame does not necessarily mean letting yourself off
the hook if you have done something wrong in your eyes. It does mean taking an appropriate amount of responsibility and coming to terms with whatever led you to feel this way. There are five aspects to overcoming guilt and
shame: assessing the seriousness of your actions, weighing personal responsibility, breaking the silence, making reparations for any harm you caused,
and self-forgiveness. Often only one or two of these steps are necessary to
help us overcome guilt. Overcoming deep shame may require all five steps.

Assessing the Seriousness of Actions

We can feel guilty or ashamed about both large and small actions. How would
you compare the seriousness of these three experiences?

1. Situation	2. Moods	3. Automatic Thoughts (Images)
Who? What? When? Where?	a. What did you feel? b. Rate each mood (0–100%).	a. What was going though your mind just before you started to feel this way? Any other thoughts? Images? b. Circle the hot thought.
Driving home from a restaurant after having dinner with Julie. She was talking about her father's recent visit.	Shame 100%	Image/memory of my father crawling into bed with me. I tried to pretend that I was asleep but that didn't stop him. Visual memories of the sexual abuse. I must be an awful person for this to have happened to me. I'm a despicable person. I could never tell Julie this happened. If she knew, she would think I'm terrible and would never want to be around me again.

FIGURE 12.1. Marissa's Thought Record: Shame.

1. Toby was tired at the end of the day. Her phone rang and she decided not to answer it because she didn't feel like talking to anyone. She heard her mother's voice on the answering machine saying, "Toby, are you there? I want to tell you about my vacation." Toby didn't answer the phone.

2. After Toby's mother had left her message, the phone rang again. When Toby heard her best friend's voice on the answering machine, she picked up the phone and chatted for 10 minutes.

3. The next day Toby told her mother that she had not been home when her mother called the night before.

Toby's three experiences describe fairly small events. Yet many people would judge the seriousness of these events differently. For which of these three events would you be likely to feel guilty? Why?

Your evaluation of the seriousness of an action or thought depends on your own internal rules and values. Many people say that they would feel more guilty about the direct lie in the third Toby example than about not answering the phone in the first example. Some people say that they would feel equally guilty in all three examples.

Frequent guilt and shame either mean that you are living your life in a way that violates your principles (e.g., having an affair when you believe in monogamous marriage) or that you are judging too many small actions as serious. To evaluate the seriousness of your actions leading to guilt and shame, you can complete a Thought Record as you learned to do in Chapters 4–7 and weigh all the evidence to see if your behavior or thoughts warrant the degree of guilt or shame you are feeling.

The Hint Box on the next page lists questions you can ask yourself to assess the seriousness of your actions. These questions encourage you to look at the situation from different perspectives. This will be particularly helpful if you tend to feel guilt or shame in many situations, even when others with similar values do not feel that way. Perspective-shifting questions can help evaluate the seriousness of your actions. Ask yourself, "How important will this seem in five years?" Having an affair will almost certainly still seem like a big violation of a monogamous relationship in five years. Arriving home late for dinner three nights in a row will not seem important in five years, even if it is a distressing event for you or your partner now. Therefore, lasting guilt about an affair would make more sense than lasting guilt about arriving home late for dinner.

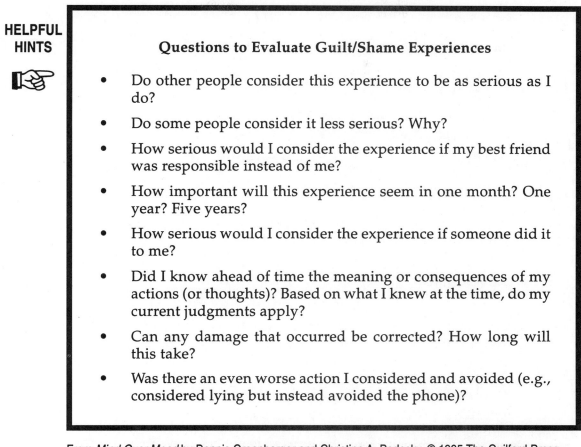

HELPFUL HINTS ☞

Questions to Evaluate Guilt/Shame Experiences

- Do other people consider this experience to be as serious as I do?

- Do some people consider it less serious? Why?

- How serious would I consider the experience if my best friend was responsible instead of me?

- How important will this experience seem in one month? One year? Five years?

- How serious would I consider the experience if someone did it to me?

- Did I know ahead of time the meaning or consequences of my actions (or thoughts)? Based on what I knew at the time, do my current judgments apply?

- Can any damage that occurred be corrected? How long will this take?

- Was there an even worse action I considered and avoided (e.g., considered lying but instead avoided the phone)?

From *Mind Over Mood* by Dennis Greenberger and Christine A. Padesky. © 1995 The Guilford Press.

Weighing Personal Responsibility

Once you have assessed the seriousness of your actions, it is helpful to weigh how much of the violation is your sole, personal responsibility. Marissa felt ashamed that she was molested as a child. The molestation was certainly a serious event in her life, but was she responsible for it? Vic felt guilty that he blew up in anger at his wife, Judy, one night when she started complaining about their overdue credit card bills. Was he responsible for his angry reaction?

A good way to weigh personal responsibility is to construct a "responsibility pie." To do this, list all the people and aspects of a situation that contributed to an event about which you feel guilty or ashamed. Include yourself on the list. Then draw a pie and assign slices of the responsibility for the event in sizes that reflect relative responsibility. Draw your own slice last so that you do not prematurely assign too much responsibility to yourself.

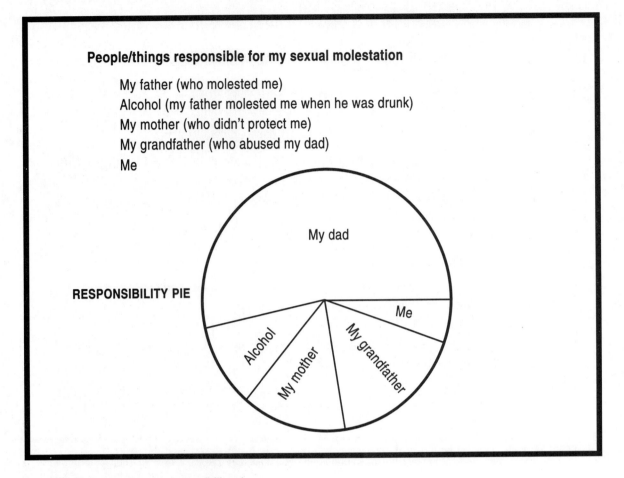

People/things responsible for my sexual molestation

My father (who molested me)
Alcohol (my father molested me when he was drunk)
My mother (who didn't protect me)
My grandfather (who abused my dad)
Me

RESPONSIBILITY PIE

FIGURE 12.2. Marissa's responsibility pie.

Figure 12.2 shows what people and things Marissa identified as partly responsible for her sexual molestation and how she completed her first responsibility pie. Although Marissa had always felt personally responsible for being molested, she learned that her part of the responsibility was actually very small. She decided that she felt responsible only for not saying no to her dad. Most of the responsibility for what happened was her father's, and even the slices representing her mother, grandfather, and alcohol were larger than Marissa's.

When Marissa showed her responsibility pie to her therapist, they discussed further her "responsibility" for the molestation. After a number of sessions, Marissa came to understand and believe that she was not at all responsible for being molested. She learned that molestation is entirely an adult responsibility; like most children, she did not have the knowledge or security to say no at age 6 or even at age 13. When she did finally say no at age 14, the molestation stopped. But stopping her father at age 14 did not mean that she had the ability to do this all along. Her father may have been unwilling to risk confrontation with her as an older child. But he would have had no trouble overpowering her when she was younger. Even if she had said no when she was younger, it probably would not have stopped him. The responsibility pie helped Marissa resolve her guilt.

Vic completed a responsibility pie (Figure 12.3) when he felt guilty about blowing up at Judy when she complained to him about overdue credit card bills. His anger was a serious violation of his promise to Judy that he would not attack her in anger. Although he did not hit or shove Judy, he physically intimidated her by standing close to her and shouting in her face.

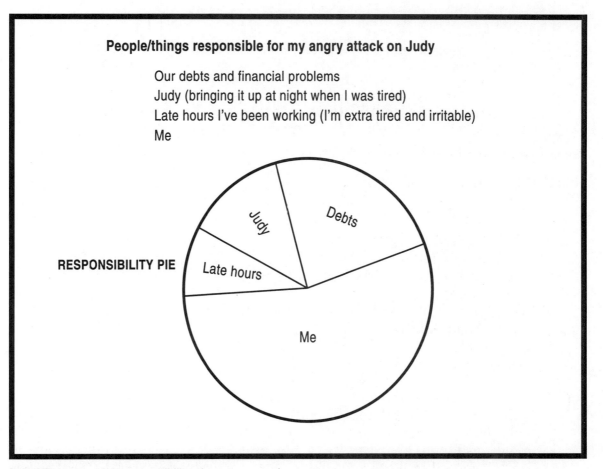

People/things responsible for my angry attack on Judy

Our debts and financial problems
Judy (bringing it up at night when I was tired)
Late hours I've been working (I'm extra tired and irritable)
Me

RESPONSIBILITY PIE

Judy

Debts

Late hours

Me

FIGURE 12.3. Vic's responsibility pie.

As you see, Vic decided that he was primarily responsible for his anger outburst. Although Judy, their debts, and his late work hours contributed to his anger, he felt that he could have handled the situation in a less intimidating fashion. Therefore, Vic decided that he should make reparations to Judy for what he had done and to work to change his anger response.

As the Marissa and Vic examples illustrate, responsibility pies can help you evaluate the levels of responsibility of each of the contributors to a situation. People who often feel guilty over small things find that responsibility pies help them recognize that they are not 100% responsible for the undesirable things that happen. People who feel guilt or shame when they have caused harm to others can use a responsibility pie to evaluate their role in any damage that was done before making reparations.

EXERCISE: Using a Responsibility Pie for Guilt or Shame

(1) Think of a negative event or situation in your life for which you think you are responsible (and, therefore, feel guilt or shame). (2) List below all the people and circumstances which could have contributed to the outcome. Place yourself on the bottom of the list. (3) Starting at the top of your list, divide the pie below into slices, labeling these slices with the names of the people or circumstances on your list. Assign bigger pieces to people or circumstances which you think have greater responsibility for the event or situation examined. (4) When you are finished, notice how much responsibility is yours alone and how much you share with others.

WORKSHEET 12.2: Using a Responsibility Pie for Guilt or Shame

1. Negative event or situation leading to guilt or shame:_____

2. People and circumstances which could have contributed to this outcome:

_____

_____

_____

_____

_____

_____

_____

_____

_____

_____

3.

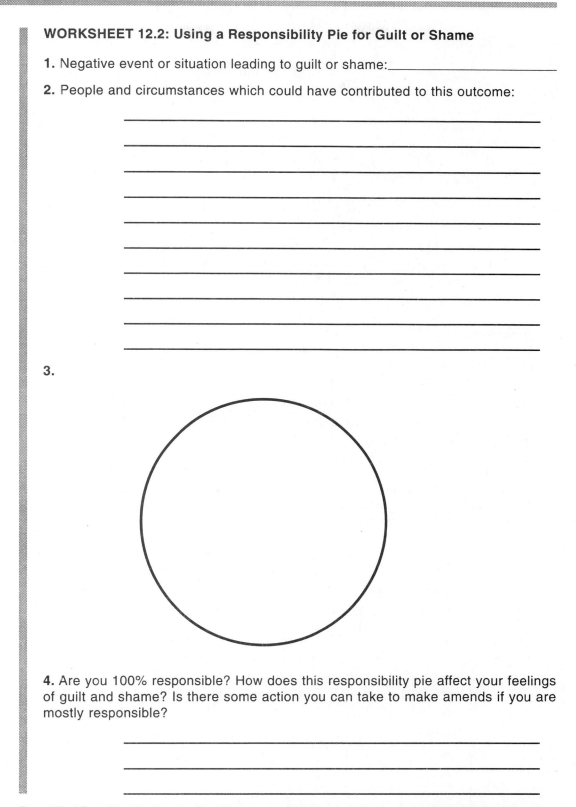

4. Are you 100% responsible? How does this responsibility pie affect your feelings of guilt and shame? Is there some action you can take to make amends if you are mostly responsible?

_____

_____

_____

Breaking the Silence

When secretiveness surrounds shame, it may be important to talk to a trusted person about what occurred. The need to keep silent is often based on the anticipation that revealing the secret will result in condemnation, criticism, or rejection by others. It is not unusual for people who have carried a secret for a lifetime to be surprised at the acceptance they receive when they reveal their secret. Acceptance runs counter to the anticipated rejection and forces a reassessment of the meaning of the secret.

Although you may not trust anyone fully, it is important to reveal your secret to the people you trust the most. You may tell people how anxious it makes you feel to reveal your secret and how difficult it is for you to do. Be sure to talk to someone when you will have adequate time to say everything you need to say and to talk about the feedback you get.

Self-Forgiveness

Being a good person doesn't mean that you will never do any bad things. Part of being human is making mistakes. If, after careful evaluation, you conclude that you have done some things wrong, then self-forgiveness may help alleviate some of your guilt or shame.

No one is perfect. All of us, at one point or another, have violated our own principles or standards. We feel guilty and ashamed if we believe that what we did means that we are bad. But violations do not necessarily mean that we are bad. Our actions may have been linked to a particular situation or to a specific time in our lives.

Self-forgiveness results in a change in interpretation of the meaning of the violation or mistake we made. Our understanding may change from "I made this mistake because I'm an awful person" to "I made this mistake during an awful time in my life when I didn't care if I behaved this way" or from "I was abused because I deserved it" to "I was abused because my parents were out-of-control alcoholics." Self-forgiveness also involves recognizing your own imperfections and mistakes and accepting yourself, shortcomings and all, and recognizing that life has not been one mistake or violation after another. Self-forgiveness includes recognizing our good and bad qualities, our strengths as well as weaknesses, assets as well as liabilities.

Making Reparations

If you have injured another person, it is important to make amends for your actions. Asking to repair the damage you have done can be an important component in healing yourself and the relationship. Making amends involves recognizing your transgression, being courageous enough to face the person you have hurt, asking forgiveness, and determining what you can do to repair the hurt you caused.

CHAPTER 12 SUMMARY

- Anger is characterized by muscle tension, increased heart rate, increased blood pressure, and defensiveness or attack.

- The cognitive component of anger involves the perception of being mistreated or perceiving others as being hurtful or unfair.

- Anger can range from mild irritation to rage.

- Methods that are effective in controlling anger include cognitive restructuring, preparing for events in which you are at high risk for experiencing anger, imagery, recognizing the early warning signs of anger, timeouts, assertion training, and couples therapy.

- We feel guilty when we believe that we have done something wrong.

- Guilt is often accompanied by thoughts containing the words "should" and "ought."

- Shame involves the perception that we have done something wrong, that we need to keep it a secret, and that what we have done means something terrible about us.

- Guilt and shame can be lessened or eliminated by assessing the seriousness of your actions, weighing personal responsibility, breaking the silence, self-forgiveness, and making reparations.

Epilogue

A wise Chinese fisherman, while fishing off the end of a pier, was approached by a hungry woman who hadn't eaten anything for several days. Eyeing the basket of fish he had caught, the woman begged him to give her some fish to satisfy her hunger. After thinking for a moment, the fisherman replied, "I'm not going to give you any of my fish, but if you sit down next to me for awhile and pick up a pole, I'll teach you how to fish. That way you will not only eat today, you will learn how to feed yourself for the rest of your life." The woman took the fisherman's advice, learned to fish, and never went hungry again.

This metaphor suggests that *Mind Over Mood* can help you today and in the future. Like the hungry woman, you have learned skills that, if practiced, will help you for the rest of your life.

You have followed the treatment and progress of Ben, Linda, Marissa, and Vic throughout this book. This epilogue describes what happened to these four people as time went by.

BEN: *Older and better.*

Ben conquered his depression by testing his thoughts on Thought Records and by doing experiments to learn new ways of interacting with his children

208

and grandchildren. By the end of therapy he felt much happier and resumed golfing with his friends, tinkering with projects in his garage, and doing a variety of activities with his wife, Sylvie. In addition, Ben and Sylvie talked about how they would each cope if the other died. While Ben hoped Sylvie would live as long as he, he felt more certain that he could learn to enjoy his life even if she died first.

The dramatic improvement in his mood pleased and surprised Ben. He sprang up from his chair at the end of his last therapy session and gave his therapist a firm handshake, "Thank you, doctor. You've been a terrific help and you know I didn't believe therapy could help." Ben's therapist smiled and told Ben, "Well, you deserve the credit. You worked very hard to feel better."

Ben had worked hard in therapy. Almost every day he made some at-

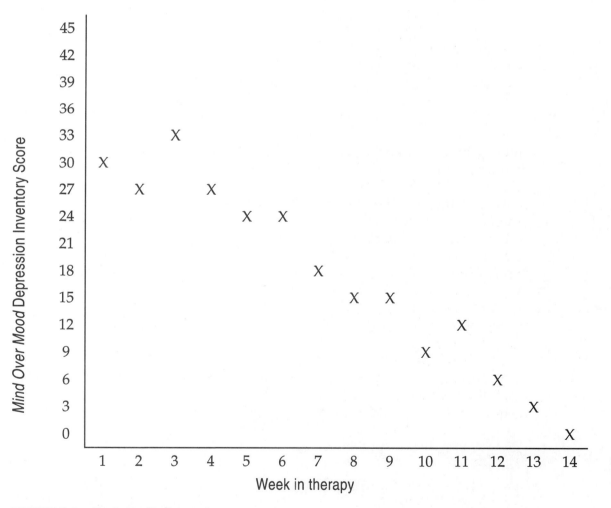

FIGURE E.1. Ben's weekly depression scores.

tempt to feel better. Some days he identified feelings and thoughts; other days he increased his positive activities or experimented with new behaviors. Even with this consistent effort, Ben's improvement varied from week to week. Figure E.1, at the bottom of page 209, shows Ben's depression chart for the time he was in therapy.

Notice that Ben might have thought he wasn't making any progress in week 4 when his depression scores were mostly unchanged. But over time, Ben's depression decreased, especially after week 6 when he began to use Thought Records. Even though Ben's depression scores sometimes increased or stayed the same, over time, he felt better.

MARISSA: *Finally my life seems worth living.*

As you see on Marissa's depression chart (Figure E.2 on the following page), her improvement pattern was quite different from Ben's.

Marissa continued in therapy for several months, and her depression went up and down throughout this time period. During particularly difficult times (e.g., when she was getting critical feedback at work, when she and her therapist were discussing her childhood abuse, when Marissa became discouraged and stopped doing Thought Records) her depression scores were higher (she was more depressed). When Marissa had greater success with problem solving, Thought Records, and experiments, her depression scores were lower (she was less depressed).

At times, Marissa's depression scores were as high as when she started therapy, but notice that her scores were mostly lower in the later weeks of her chart. In the first ten weeks, Marissa's depression scores were above 30 for seven weeks. In the next ten weeks, Marissa's scores were above 30 for only four weeks. In the next ten weeks her scores were above 30 in only one week. So, although Marissa continued to struggle with depression for months, her chart helped her see that she had fewer very depressed weeks as she practiced using Thought Records and the other skills she learned.

Marissa has now been using the techniques described in this manual for over three years. She is using the methods on her own now, although she goes back to see her therapist to problem solve when she feels stuck. Marissa has not made any suicide attempts in the past two and one-half years. She no longer feels guilty or ashamed about her childhood abuse history. She has done well in her job and has received positive evaluations from her supervisor. Her second child has entered college, and with both children living away from home, Marissa moved to a smaller apartment in a building where she could keep a garden. Marissa is living alone for the first time in her life. She's made some new friends and feels more hope for the future.

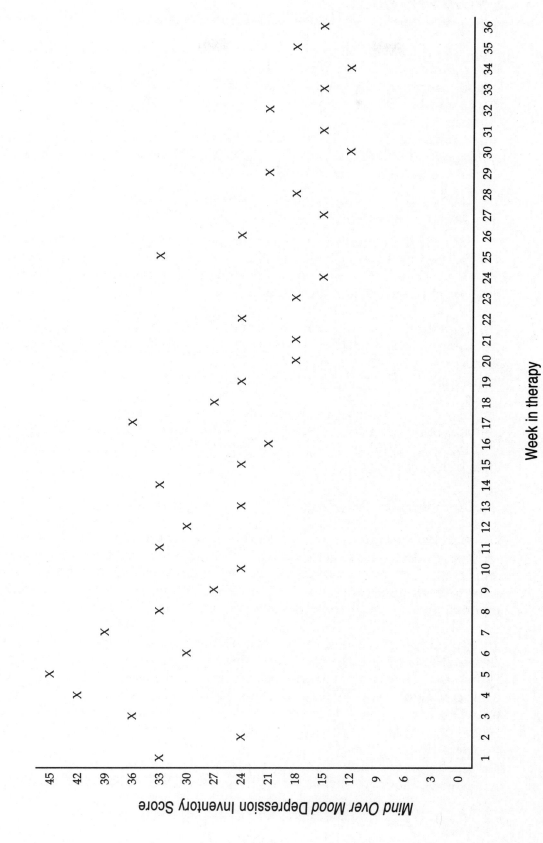

FIGURE E.2. Marissa's weekly depression scores.

LINDA: *Frequent flyer.*

As you learned in Chapter 8, Linda was successful in overcoming her panic attacks and her fear of flying. Three key steps led to her success.

1. Linda identified the physical sensations (e.g., rapid heart rate) that frightened her and the catastrophic fears (e.g., "I'm having a heart attack") attached to these sensations.

2. With the help of her therapist, Linda constructed alternative explanations for these sensations (e.g., anxiety, excitement, coffee).

3. Linda did a number of experiments to gather information and to test whether her catastrophic beliefs or alternative explanations matched her life experiences better. These experiments were done in the therapist's office, in imagery, at home, and on airplanes.

Over time, Linda became confident that the physical sensations she experienced were fueled by anxiety, not physical danger. She learned and practiced a number of strategies for reducing her anxiety. She was flying with comfort a few months after beginning therapy.

Linda kept the job promotion and became regional supervisor for her company. She used the skills she learned in therapy for identifying and modifying thoughts and feelings to help her manage the additional pressures of her new job.

VIC: *The perfect solution—to be OK.*

Vic initially went into treatment wanting to feel more confident, to feel better about himself, and to get help in maintaining his sobriety. As time passed, some of Vic's therapy goals changed. He remained steadfast in his commitment to sobriety. However, he began to realize that he had problems with anger, depression, and anxiety that were threatening his marriage.

Vic addressed each of these issues in turn. His progress was characterized by hard work, sustained effort, and steady improvement interrupted by two episodes of binge drinking and significant deterioration in his life. After completing approximately 35 Thought Records, Vic developed a good ability to identify and alter his dysfunctional thoughts. Thought Records helped Vic control his urges to drink and minimized the frequency of his angry outbursts.

Vic used the Core Belief Record (Worksheet 9.5) to assess his beliefs of inadequacy and the new Core Belief Record (Worksheet 9.6) to record evidence supporting his new sense of adequacy and self-worth (Figures E.3 and E.4).

CORE BELIEF: *I am inadequate.*

Evidence or experiences that suggest that the core belief is not true 100% of the time:

1. *My children love me.*

2. *My wife loves me.*

3. *My children have turned out well, and I have had some part in that.*

4. *I have friends and acceptance at my church.*

5. *At times I believe I am doing well at my job.*

6. *Customers like me.*

7. *I am able to maintain long-term relationships with most of my accounts.*

8. *I have gone for long periods of time without drinking.*

9. *I am getting better at controlling my angry outbursts.*

10. *My relationship with Judy is getting closer and better.*

11. *Most of the time I am a good father.*

12. *My boss tells me that overall I am successfully managing my territory.*

FIGURE E.3. Vic's Core Belief Record.

NEW BELIEF: *I am competent*

Evidence or experiences that support new belief:

1. *My daughter and I visited a college she was considering attending. I helped her get acquainted and ask questions. She told me she appreciated my help.*

2. *I helped my son with a science project he was working on. I didn't do it for him, but I helped him think it through in a way that helped him.*

3. *Judy expressed admiration for my continuing sobriety.*

4. *I sold products to four new accounts last month.*

5. *I was asked by the minister at my church to help organize meetings for new church members.*

6. *I attended an AA meeting Tuesday night when I felt like drinking.*

7. *I got my monthly reports in on time.*

8. *I stayed calm when Judy and I were discussing our bills.*

FIGURE E.4.   Vic's new Core Belief Record.

After his second episode of binge drinking, Vic was successfully able to control his urges to drink and maintain his sobriety. He attributes his sobriety to being able to recognize and alter the thoughts and beliefs that accompany his urges to drink.

Vic and Judy decided that couples therapy would be beneficial. Couples therapy taught them how to improve their communication and express their feelings clearly. The improved communication allowed Judy and Vic to assess the accuracy of their perceptions. Further, therapy helped Vic and Judy repair their trust, which had been weakened by years of anger.

As his therapy was coming to an end, Vic realized that he would continue to face challenges on a daily basis. As part of his relapse prevention plan, Vic decided to do two Thought Records per week. He also decided to continue gathering data on his new Core Belief Record to support his new sense of self-worth and adequacy, rather than trying to be perfect. Vic attributes his ongoing sobriety, improved marriage, and increased sense of happiness to these strategies and methods.

The Prologue to *Mind Over Mood* described how an oyster turns an irritant into a valuable pearl. Our hope is that *Mind Over Mood* has helped you learn new skills to transform irritants and problems in your own life into new coping strategies and strengths. You are now more capable of evaluating your thoughts, managing your moods and changing your life. We hope that you have resolved the problems that led you to *Mind Over Mood* and that in that resolution you have gained insight, understanding, skills, and methods to transform future irritants into pearls.

Appendix

THOUGHT RECORD

1. Situation	2. Moods	3. Automatic Thoughts (Images)	4. Evidence That Supports the Hot Thought	5. Evidence That Does Not Support the Hot Thought	6. Alternative/ Balanced Thoughts	7. Rate Moods Now
Who were you with? What were you doing? When was it? Where were you?	Describe each mood in one word. Rate intensity of mood (0– 100%).	**Answer some or all of the following questions:** What was going through my mind just before I started to feel this way? What does this say about me? What does this mean about me? my life? my future? What am I afraid might happen? What is the worst thing that could happen if this is true? What does this mean about how the other person(s) feel(s)/think(s) about me? What does this mean about the other person(s) or people in general? What images or memories do I have in this situation?	Circle hot thought in previous column for which you are looking for evidence. Write factual evidence to support this conclusion. (Try to avoid mind-reading and interpretation of facts.)	Ask yourself the questions in the Hint Box (p. 70) to help discover evidence which does not support your hot thought.	Ask yourself the questions in the Hint Box (p. 95) to generate alternative or balanced thoughts. Write an alternative or balanced thought. Rate how much you believe in each alternative or balanced thought (0– 100%).	Copy the feelings from Column 2. Rerate the intensity of each feeling from 0 to 100% as well as any new records.

From *Mind Over Mood* by Dennis Greenberger and Christine A. Padesky. © 1995 The Guilford Press.

THOUGHT RECORD

1. Situation	2. Moods	3. Automatic Thoughts (Images)	4. Evidence That Supports the Hot Thought	5. Evidence That Does Not Support the Hot Thought	6. Alternative/ Balanced Thoughts	7. Rate Moods Now
Who were you with? What were you doing? When was it? Where were you?	Describe each mood in one word. Rate intensity of mood (0–100%).	**Answer some or all of the following questions:** What was going through my mind just before I started to feel this way? What does this say about me? What does this mean about me? my life? my future? What am I afraid might happen? What is the worst thing that could happen if this is true? What does this mean about how the other person(s) feel(s)/think(s) about me? What does this mean about the other person(s) or people in general? What images or memories do I have in this situation?	Circle hot thought in previous column for which you are looking for evidence. Write factual evidence to support this conclusion. (Try to avoid mind-reading and interpretation of facts.)	Ask yourself the questions in the Hint Box (p. 70) to help discover evidence which does not support your hot thought.	Ask yourself the questions in the Hint Box (p. 95) *to* generate alternative or balanced thoughts. Write an alternative or balanced thought. Rate how much you believe in each alternative or balanced thought (0–100%).	Copy the feelings from Column 2. Rerate the intensity of each feeling from 0 to 100% as well as any new records.

THOUGHT RECORD

1. Situation	2. Moods	3. Automatic Thoughts (Images)	4. Evidence That Supports the Hot Thought	5. Evidence That Does Not Support the Hot Thought	6. Alternative/ Balanced Thoughts	7. Rate Moods Now
Who were you with? What were you doing? When was it? Where were you?	Describe each mood in one word. Rate intensity of mood (0–100%).	**Answer some or all of the following questions:** What was going through my mind just before I started to feel this way? What does this say about me? What does this mean about me? my life? my future? What am I afraid might happen? What is the worst thing that could happen if this is true? What does this mean about how the other person(s) feel(s)/think(s) about me? What does this mean about the other person(s) or people in general? What images or memories do I have in this situation?	Circle hot thought in previous column for which you are looking for evidence. Write factual evidence to support this conclusion. (Try to avoid mind-reading and interpretation of facts.)	Ask yourself the questions in the Hint Box (p. 70) to help discover evidence which does not support your hot thought.	Ask yourself the questions in the Hint Box (p. 95) to generate alternative or balanced thoughts. Write an alternative or balanced thought. Rate how much you believe in each alternative or balanced thought (0–100%).	Copy the feelings from Column 2. Rerate the intensity of each feeling from 0 to 100% as well as any new records.

From *Mind Over Mood* by Dennis Greenberger and Christine A. Padesky. © 1995 The Guilford Press.

THOUGHT RECORD

1. Situation	2. Moods	3. Automatic Thoughts (Images)	4. Evidence That Supports the Hot Thought	5. Evidence That Does Not Support the Hot Thought	6. Alternative/ Balanced Thoughts	7. Rate Moods Now
Who were you with? What were you doing? When was it? Where were you?	Describe each mood in one word. Rate intensity of mood (0–100%).	**Answer some or all of the following questions:** What was going through my mind just before I started to feel this way? What does this say about me? What does this mean about me? my life? my future? What am I afraid might happen? What is the worst thing that could happen if this is true? What does this mean about how the other person(s) feel(s)/think(s) about me? What does this mean about the other person(s) or people in general? What images or memories do I have in this situation?	Circle hot thought in previous column for which you are looking for evidence. Write factual evidence to support this conclusion. (Try to avoid mind-reading and interpretation of facts.)	Ask yourself the questions in the Hint Box (p. 70) to help discover evidence which does not support your hot thought.	Ask yourself the questions in the Hint Box (p. 95) to generate alternative or balanced thoughts. Write an alternative or balanced thought. Rate how much you believe in each alternative or balanced thought (0–100%).	Copy the feelings from Column 2. Rerate the intensity of each feeling from 0 to 100% as well as any new records.

THOUGHT RECORD

1. Situation	2. Moods	3. Automatic Thoughts (Images)	4. Evidence That Supports the Hot Thought	5. Evidence That Does Not Support the Hot Thought	6. Alternative/ Balanced Thoughts	7. Rate Moods Now
Who were you with? What were you doing? When was it? Where were you?	Describe each mood in one word. Rate intensity of mood (0–100%).	**Answer some or all of the following questions:** What was going through my mind just before I started to feel this way? What does this say about me? What does this mean about me? my life? my future? What am I afraid might happen? What is the worst thing that could happen if this is true? What does this mean about how the other person(s) feel(s)/think(s) about me? What does this mean about the other person(s) or people in general? What images or memories do I have in this situation?	Circle hot thought in previous column for which you are looking for evidence. Write factual evidence to support this conclusion. (Try to avoid mind-reading and interpretation of facts.)	Ask yourself the questions in the Hint Box (p. 70) to help discover evidence which does not support your hot thought.	Ask yourself the questions in the Hint Box (p. 95) to generate alternative or balanced thoughts. Write an alternative or balanced thought. Rate how much you believe in each alternative or balanced thought (0–100%).	Copy the feelings from Column 2. Rerate the intensity of each feeling from 0 to 100% as well as any new records.

THOUGHT RECORD

1. Situation	2. Moods	3. Automatic Thoughts (Images)	4. Evidence That Supports the Hot Thought	5. Evidence That Does Not Support the Hot Thought	6. Alternative/ Balanced Thoughts	7. Rate Moods Now
Who were you with? What were you doing? When was it? Where were you?	Describe each mood in one word. Rate intensity of mood (0—100%).	**Answer some or all of the following questions:** What was going through my mind just before I started to feel this way? What does this say about me? What does this mean about me? my life? my future? What am I afraid might happen? What is the worst thing that could happen if this is true? What does this mean about how the other person(s) feel(s)/think(s) about me? What does this mean about the other person(s) or people in general? What images or memories do I have in this situation?	Circle hot thought in previous column for which you are looking for evidence. Write factual evidence to support this conclusion. (Try to avoid mind-reading and interpretation of facts.)	Ask yourself the questions in the Hint Box (p. 70) to help discover evidence which does not support your hot thought.	Ask yourself the questions in the Hint Box (p. 95) to generate alternative or balanced thoughts. Write an alternative or balanced thought. Rate how much you believe in each alternative or balanced thought (0—100%).	Copy the feelings from Column 2. Rerate the intensity of each feeling from 0 to 100% as well as any new records.

THOUGHT RECORD

1. Situation	2. Moods	3. Automatic Thoughts (Images)	4. Evidence That Supports the Hot Thought	5. Evidence That Does Not Support the Hot Thought	6. Alternative/ Balanced Thoughts	7. Rate Moods Now
Who were you with? What were you doing? When was it? Where were you?	Describe each mood in one word. Rate intensity of mood (0–100%).	**Answer some or all of the following questions:** What was going through my mind just before I started to feel this way? What does this say about me? What does this mean about me? my life? my future? What am I afraid might happen? What is the worst thing that could happen if this is true? What does this mean about how the other person(s) feel(s)/think(s) about me? What does this mean about the other person(s) or people in general? What images or memories do I have in this situation?	Circle hot thought in previous column for which you are looking for evidence. Write factual evidence to support this conclusion. (Try to avoid mind-reading and interpretation of facts.)	Ask yourself the questions in the Hint Box (p. 70) to help discover evidence which does not support your hot thought.	Ask yourself the questions in the Hint Box (p. 95) *to* generate alternative or balanced thoughts. Write an alternative or balanced thought. Rate how much you believe in each alternative or balanced thought (0–100%).	Copy the feelings from Column 2. Rerate the intensity of each feeling from 0 to 100% as well as any new records.

THOUGHT RECORD

1. Situation	2. Moods	3. Automatic Thoughts (Images)	4. Evidence That Supports the Hot Thought	5. Evidence That Does Not Support the Hot Thought	6. Alternative/ Balanced Thoughts	7. Rate Moods Now
Who were you with? What were you doing? When was it? Where were you?	Describe each mood in one word. Rate intensity of mood (0–100%).	**Answer some or all of the following questions:** What was going through my mind just before I started to feel this way? What does this say about me? What does this mean about me? my life? my future? What am I afraid might happen? What is the worst thing that could happen if this is true? What does this mean about how the other person(s) feel(s)/think(s) about me? What does this mean about the other person(s) or people in general? What images or memories do I have in this situation?	Circle hot thought in previous column for which you are looking for evidence. Write factual evidence to support this conclusion. (Try to avoid mind-reading and interpretation of facts.)	Ask yourself the questions in the Hint Box (p. 70) to help discover evidence which does not support your hot thought.	Ask yourself the questions in the Hint Box (p. 95) to generate alternative or balanced thoughts. Write an alternative or balanced thought. Rate how much you believe in each alternative or balanced thought (0–100%).	Copy the feelings from Column 2. Rerate the intensity of each feeling from 0 to 100% as well as any new records.

THOUGHT RECORD

1. Situation	2. Moods	3. Automatic Thoughts (Images)	4. Evidence That Supports the Hot Thought	5. Evidence That Does Not Support the Hot Thought	6. Alternative/ Balanced Thoughts	7. Rate Moods Now
Who were you with? What were you doing? When was it? Where were you?	Describe each mood in one word. Rate intensity of mood (0–100%).	**Answer some or all of the following questions:** What was going through my mind just before I started to feel this way? What does this say about me? What does this mean about me? my life? my future? What am I afraid might happen? What is the worst thing that could happen if this is true? What does this mean about how the other person(s) feel(s)/think(s) about me? What does this mean about the other person(s) or people in general? What images or memories do I have in this situation?	Circle hot thought in previous column for which you are looking for evidence. Write factual evidence to support this conclusion. (Try to avoid mind-reading and interpretation of facts.)	Ask yourself the questions in the Hint Box (p. 70) to help discover evidence which does not support your hot thought.	Ask yourself the questions in the Hint Box (p. 95) to generate alternative or balanced thoughts. Write an alternative or balanced thought. Rate how much you believe in each alternative or balanced thought (0–100%).	Copy the feelings from Column 2. Rerate the intensity of each feeling from 0 to 100% as well as any new records.

THOUGHT TO BE TESTED: _____

_____

_____

Experiment	Prediction	Possible problems	Strategies to overcome these problems	Outcome of experiment	How much does the outcome support the thought that was tested? (0–100%)

WHAT HAVE I LEARNED FROM THESE EXPERIMENTS? _____

_____

_____

_____

THOUGHT TO BE TESTED: _____

_____

_____

Experiment	Prediction	Possible problems	Strategies to overcome these problems	Outcome of experiment	How much does the outcome support the thought that was tested? (0–100%)

WHAT HAVE I LEARNED FROM THESE EXPERIMENTS? _____

_____

_____

WORKSHEET 8.2: Action Plan

GOAL:_____

Action plan	Time to begin	Possible problems	Strategies to overcome problems	Progress

WORKSHEET 8.2: Action Plan

GOAL:_____

Action plan	Time to begin	Possible problems	Strategies to overcome problems	Progress

WORKSHEET 9.6. Core Belief Record: Recording Evidence That Supports an Alternative Core Belief

Write out an alternative core belief that explains the experiences you recorded on Worksheet 9.5. Then begin recording small events and experiences that support the new core belief. Over the next few months, continue to write down experiences that support your new belief.

New Core Belief: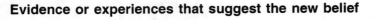

Evidence or experiences that suggest the new belief

1. _____
2. _____
3. _____
4. _____
5. _____
6. _____
7. _____
8. _____
9. _____
10. _____
11. _____
12. _____
13. _____
14. _____
15. _____
16. _____
17. _____
18. _____
19. _____
20. _____
21. _____
22. _____
23. _____
24. _____
25. _____

WORKSHEET 9.7: Rating Confidence in a New Core Belief

On the first line of Worksheet 9.7, write the new core belief you developed for Worksheet 9.6. Then enter the date and rate the new core belief by placing an "X" on the scale above the number that best matches how much you think this new belief is true. To measure your progress in strengthening your new core belief, rerate the new core belief every few weeks.

New core belief: _____

Ratings of confidence in the belief

Date: _____

0	25	50	75	100

Date: _____

0	25	50	75	100

Date: _____

0	25	50	75	100

Date: _____

0	25	50	75	100

Date: _____

0	25	50	75	100

Date: _____

0	25	50	75	100

Date: _____

0	25	50	75	100

WORKSHEET 9.8: Rating Personal Experiences

Situation:_____ Quality I am rating:_____

0	25	50	75	100

Situation:_____ Quality I am rating:_____

0	25	50	75	100

Situation:_____ Quality I am rating:_____

0	25	50	75	100

Situation:_____ Quality I am rating:_____

0	25	50	75	100

Situation:_____ Quality I am rating:_____

0	25	50	75	100

Situation:_____ Quality I am rating:_____

0	25	50	75	100

Summary:_____

_____

_____

_____

_____

_____

_____

WORKSHEET 9.9: Historical Test of New Core Belief

NEW CORE BELIEF: _____

Age	Experiences I had that are consistent with the new core belief
Birth–2	
3–5	
6–12	
13–18	
19–25	
26–35	
36–50	
51–65	
66+	

SUMMARY: _____

_____

_____

_____

WORKSHEET 10.1: *Mind Over Mood* Depression Inventory

In order to use this inventory multiple times, do not write on this page. Indicate on the answer sheet on the following page the numbered answer that best describes how much you have experienced each symptom over the last week.

	Not at all	Sometimes	Frequently	Most of the time
1. Sad or depressed mood	0	1	2	3
2. Feeling guilty	0	1	2	3
3. Irritable mood	0	1	2	3
4. Less interest or pleasure in usual activities	0	1	2	3
5. Withdraw from or avoid people	0	1	2	3
6. Find it harder than usual to do things	0	1	2	3
7. See myself as worthless	0	1	2	3
8. Trouble concentrating	0	1	2	3
9. Difficulty making decisions	0	1	2	3
10. Suicidal thoughts	0	1	2	3
11. Recurrent thoughts of death	0	1	2	3
12. Spend time thinking about a suicide plan	0	1	2	3
13. Low self-esteem	0	1	2	3
14. See the future as hopeless	0	1	2	3
15. Self-critical thoughts	0	1	2	3
16. Tiredness or loss of energy	0	1	2	3
17. Significant weight loss or decrease in appetite (do not include weight loss from a diet plan)	0	1	2	3
18. Change in sleep pattern—difficulty sleeping or sleeping more or less than usual	0	1	2	3
19. Decreased sexual desire	0	1	2	3

Score (of total circled numbers)

Mind Over Mood Depression Inventory Answer Sheet

In each blank, write your numerical answer reflecting how much you have experienced each symptom listed on the previous page over the last week. Total your score and record this score and the date you took this test on the graph on page 156.

Item	Item	Item	Item	Item
1. _____	1. _____	1. _____	1. _____	1. _____
2. _____	2. _____	2. _____	2. _____	2. _____
3. _____	3. _____	3. _____	3. _____	3. _____
4. _____	4. _____	4. _____	4. _____	4. _____
5. _____	5. _____	5. _____	5. _____	5. _____
6. _____	6. _____	6. _____	6. _____	6. _____
7. _____	7. _____	7. _____	7. _____	7. _____
8. _____	8. _____	8. _____	8. _____	8. _____
9. _____	9. _____	9. _____	9. _____	9. _____
10. _____	10. _____	10. _____	10. _____	10. _____
11. _____	11. _____	11. _____	11. _____	11. _____
12. _____	12. _____	12. _____	12. _____	12. _____
13. _____	13. _____	13. _____	13. _____	13. _____
14. _____	14. _____	14. _____	14. _____	14. _____
15. _____	15. _____	15. _____	15. _____	15. _____
16. _____	16. _____	16. _____	16. _____	16. _____
17. _____	17. _____	17. _____	17. _____	17. _____
18. _____	18. _____	18. _____	18. _____	18. _____
19. _____	19. _____	19. _____	19. _____	19. _____

Total Score _____	Total Score _____	Total Score _____	Total Score _____	Total Score _____
Date _____	Date _____	Date _____	Date _____	Date _____

WORKSHEET 10.4: Tracking Activities—Weekly Activity Schedule

Write in each box: (1) Activity. (2) Mood ratings (0–100). (Mood I am rating: _____)

Time	MONDAY	TUESDAY	WEDNESDAY	THURSDAY	FRIDAY	SATURDAY	SUNDAY
6–7 A.M.							
7–8 A.M.							
8–9 A.M.							
9–10 A.M.							
10–11 A.M.							
11–12 P.M.							
12–1 P.M.							
1–2 P.M.							
2–3 P.M.							

3-4 P.M.					
4-5 P.M.					
5-6 P.M.					
6-7 P.M.					
7-8 P.M.					
8-9 P.M.					
9-10 P.M.					
10-11 P.M.					
11-12 A.M.					
12-1 A.M.					

WORSHEET 11.1 *Mind Over Mood* Anxiety Inventory

In order to use this inventory multiple times, do not write on this page. Indicate on the answer sheet on the following page the numbered answer that best describes how much you have experienced each symptom over the last week.

	Not at all	Sometimes	Frequently	Most of the time
1. Feeling nervous	0	1	2	3
2. Frequent worrying	0	1	2	3
3. Trembling, twitching, feeling shaky	0	1	2	3
4. Muscle tension, muscle aches, muscle soreness	0	1	2	3
5. Restlessness	0	1	2	3
6. Easily tired	0	1	2	3
7. Shortness of breath	0	1	2	3
8. Rapid heartbeat	0	1	2	3
9. Sweating not due to the heat	0	1	2	3
10. Dry mouth	0	1	2	3
11. Dizziness or light-headedness	0	1	2	3
12. Nausea, diarrhea, or stomach problems	0	1	2	3
13. Frequent urination	0	1	2	3
14. Flushes (hot flashes) or chills	0	1	2	3
15. Trouble swallowing or "lump in throat"	0	1	2	3
16. Feeling keyed up or on edge	0	1	2	3
17. Quick to startle	0	1	2	3
18. Difficulty concentrating	0	1	2	3
19. Trouble falling or staying asleep	0	1	2	3
20. Irritability	0	1	2	3
21. Avoiding places where I might be anxious	0	1	2	3
22. Frequent thoughts of danger	0	1	2	3
23. Seeing myself as unable to cope	0	1	2	3
24. Frequent thoughts that something terrible will happen	0	1	2	3

Score (of total circled numbers) ☐

Mind Over Mood Anxiety Inventory Answer Sheet

In each blank, write your numerical answer reflecting how much you have experienced each symptom listed on the previous page ove the last week. Total your score and record this score and the date you took this test on the graph on page 179.

Item	Item	Item	Item	Item
1. _____	1. _____	1. _____	1. _____	1. _____
2. _____	2. _____	2. _____	2. _____	2. _____
3. _____	3. _____	3. _____	3. _____	3. _____
4. _____	4. _____	4. _____	4. _____	4. _____
5. _____	5. _____	5. _____	5. _____	5. _____
6. _____	6. _____	6. _____	6. _____	6. _____
7. _____	7. _____	7. _____	7. _____	7. _____
8. _____	8. _____	8. _____	8. _____	8. _____
9. _____	9. _____	9. _____	9. _____	9. _____
10. _____	10. _____	10. _____	10. _____	10. _____
11. _____	11. _____	11. _____	11. _____	11. _____
12. _____	12. _____	12. _____	12. _____	12. _____
13. _____	13. _____	13. _____	13. _____	13. _____
14. _____	14. _____	14. _____	14. _____	14. _____
15. _____	15. _____	15. _____	15. _____	15. _____
16. _____	16. _____	16. _____	16. _____	16. _____
17. _____	17. _____	17. _____	17. _____	17. _____
18. _____	18. _____	18. _____	18. _____	18. _____
19. _____	19. _____	19. _____	19. _____	19. _____
20. _____	20. _____	20. _____	20. _____	20. _____
21. _____	21. _____	21. _____	21. _____	21. _____
22. _____	22. _____	22. _____	22. _____	22. _____
23. _____	23. _____	23. _____	23. _____	23. _____
24. _____	24. _____	24. _____	24. _____	24. _____

Total *Score* _____	*Total* *Score* _____	*Total* *Score* _____	*Total* *Score* _____	*Total* *Score* _____
Date _____	*Date* _____	*Date* _____	*Date* _____	*Date* _____

WORKSHEET 12.2: Using a Responsibility Pie for Guilt or Shame

(1) Think of a negative event or situation in your life for which you think you are responsible (and, therefore, feel guilt or shame). (2) List below all the people and circumstances which could have contributed to the outcome. Place yourself on the bottom of the list. (3) Starting at the top of your list, divide the pie below into slices, labeling these slices with the names of the people or circumstances on your list. Assign bigger pieces to people or circumstances which you think have greater responsibility for the event or situation examined. (4) When you are finished, notice how much responsibility is yours alone and how much you share with others.

1. Negative event or situation leading to guilt or shame: _____

2. People and circumstances which could have contributed to this outcome:

_____

_____

_____

_____

_____

_____

_____

_____

_____

_____

3.

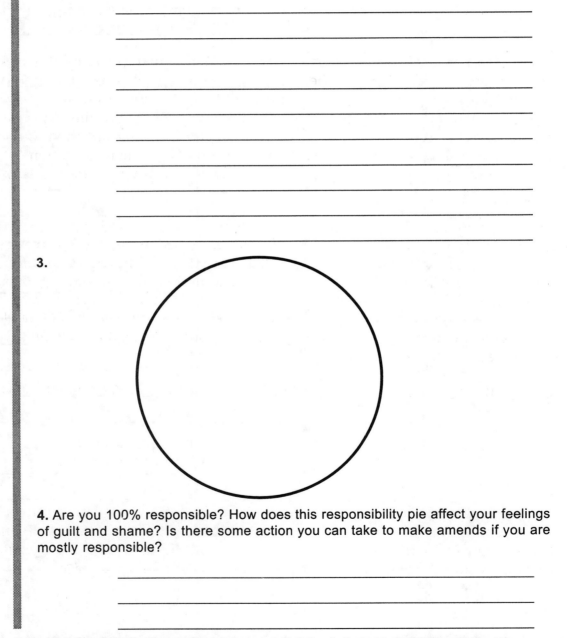

4. Are you 100% responsible? How does this responsibility pie affect your feelings of guilt and shame? Is there some action you can take to make amends if you are mostly responsible?

_____

_____

_____

Letter to Professionals

Dear Clinician:

Outcome research demonstrates the effectiveness of cognitive therapy for a wide variety of psychological problems including depression, anxiety, anger, eating disorders, substance abuse, and relationship problems. *Mind Over Mood* is a hands-on workbook that introduces the basics of cognitive therapy in a clear step-by-step format. It is designed to help readers understand their problems better and make fundamental changes in their lives with the aid of a therapist or on their own.

As a clinician, you can use *Mind Over Mood* to structure therapy, to reinforce skills taught to clients, and to continue the therapeutic learning process posttherapy. With extensive worksheets and mood questionnaires, this book actively enlists the client's participation to apply what is learned in therapy to everyday life experiences. Lessons are taught sequentially, with each chapter building on previous ones. The book's structure, along with hint boxes on how to navigate common "stuck points," helps readers successfully apply cognitive therapy principles to help resolve problems.

Available in both English and Spanish, *Mind Over Mood* can be used with individuals, couples, and groups. The book can be coordinated with cognitive therapy treatment protocols for a range of diagnoses to help clients develop specific cognitive, affective, and behavioral skills. For in-depth recommendations and troubleshooting ideas on how to incorporate this client workbook most effectively into your practice, you might wish to consult the companion volume, *Clinician's Guide to Mind Over Mood*. The order form on the next page includes more information on the *Clinician's Guide* and on the Spanish-language edition of *Mind Over Mood*.

Thank you for your interest in the *Mind Over Mood* manual. We hope it helps increase the effectiveness of the clinical services you offer.

Dennis Greenberger
Christine A. Padesky

Publisher's Note: Both *Mind Over Mood* and the *Clinician's Guide* can be purchased at better bookstores. In addition, some clinicians have opted to order multiple copies of *Mind Over Mood* to make the book readily available to clients. For details on Guilford's volume discounts, see the order form on the following page.

ORDER FORM

Also Available in Spanish!
EL CONTROL DE TU ESTADO DE ÁNIMO
MANUAL DE TRATAMIENTO DE TERAPIA COGNITIVA PARA USARIOS
(MIND OVER MOOD)
Christine A. Padesky with Dennis Greenberger
Translated by Jordi Cid

This book presents Spanish-speaking readers with the same powerful cognitive therapy tools and techniques that have made *Mind Over Mood* an acclaimed and widely used self-help resource. Expertly translated and unabridged, the book includes the full array of worksheets, questionnaires, hint boxes, and trouble-shooting guides.

256 Pages, 1998
8½" x 11" Paperback, ISBN 1-57230-358-1
Cat. #4B0358, $22.95

Plus, a Companion Book for Therapists
CLINICIAN'S GUIDE TO MIND OVER MOOD
Christine A. Padesky with Dennis Greenberger

This specially designed guide provides mental health professionals with step-by-step instructions for integrating *Mind Over Mood* into work with individuals, couples, and groups with a range of therapeutic needs. The book addresses clinicians' frequently asked questions and offers clear-cut methods for using *Mind Over Mood* as a framework for treatment, as an adjunct to treatment, or to pinpoint specific skills development.

276 Pages, 1995
Paperback, ISBN 0-89862-821-0
Cat. #4B2821, $28.00

To Order Additional Copies of MIND OVER MOOD at Quantity Discounts

If you would like to order additional copies of the English or Spanish-language edition of *Mind Over Mood* (please do not combine), see the discount schedule at right. Simply multiply the discount price times the quantity you are ordering. Add 5% of your total order for shipping. Note: Quantity discounts are available in the United States and Canada only.

Quantity	List Price	Discount	*Price Per Book
1 book	$22.95	—	$22.95
2-9 books		10% off list price	$20.66
10+ books		15% off list price	$19.51

Guilford Publications, Inc.
Promotion code 4B, 72 Spring Street, New York, NY 10012
CALL TOLL FREE (800) 365-7006
FAX: (212) 966-6708
E-mail: info@guilford.com
Website: www.guilford.com

Name

Address   Rm./Apt. No.

City   State   Zip

(   )
Daytime Phone No.

☐ Please send me a complete Guilford Catalog, Cat. #CAT.

☐ Please do not put me on your mailing list.

To order, please call the toll-free number above, order online at our website, or photocopy this coupon and mail or fax it today.

Qty	Cat. #	Title	*Price	Amount
	4B2128	**Mind Over Mood (English)**		
	4B0358	**El control de tu estado de ánimo**		
	4B2821	**Clinician's Guide to Mind Over Mood**		

* Shipping (via Priority Mail-1 to 3 weeks delivery): In U.S., add $5.00 first book, $2.50 each additional. In Canada, U.S. $7.50 first book, U.S. $2.50 each additional. Or, for quantity discount orders, add 5% of total order.

*Shipping	
Subtotal	
In NY and PA, add Sales Tax. In Canada, add G.S.T.	
TOTAL	

METHOD OF PAYMENT
☐ Check or Money Order Enclosed (U.S. Dollars only)
☐ Institutional P.O. Attached

BILL MY: ☐ MasterCard ☐ VISA ☐ American Express

Acct. #

Expiration Date

Month   Year

Signature *(Required on Credit Card Orders)*

All prices are in U.S. dollars and may be slightly higher outside the U.S. and Canada. Prices are subject to change.